Communicating
with Cancer Patients

Communicating
with Cancer Patients

John F Smyth

Endorsed by **ESMO**

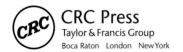

CRC Press
Taylor & Francis Group
Boca Raton   London   New York

CRC Press is an imprint of the
Taylor & Francis Group, an **informa** business

CRC Press
Taylor & Francis Group
6000 Broken Sound Parkway NW, Suite 300
Boca Raton, FL 33487-2742

© 2014 by John F. Smyth
CRC Press is an imprint of Taylor & Francis Group, an Informa business

No claim to original U.S. Government works

Printed on acid-free paper
Version Date: 20130822

International Standard Book Number-13: 978-1-4822-2678-2 (Paperback)

This book contains information obtained from authentic and highly regarded sources. While all reasonable efforts have been made to publish reliable data and information, neither the author[s] nor the publisher can accept any legal responsibility or liability for any errors or omissions that may be made. The publishers wish to make clear that any views or opinions expressed in this book by individual editors, authors or contributors are personal to them and do not necessarily reflect the views/opinions of the publishers. The information or guidance contained in this book is intended for use by medical, scientific or health-care professionals and is provided strictly as a supplement to the medical or other professional's own judgement, their knowledge of the patient's medical history, relevant manufacturer's instructions and the appropriate best practice guidelines. Because of the rapid advances in medical science, any information or advice on dosages, procedures or diagnoses should be independently verified. The reader is strongly urged to consult the drug companies' printed instructions, and their websites, before administering any of the drugs recommended in this book. This book does not indicate whether a particular treatment is appropriate or suitable for a particular individual. Ultimately it is the sole responsibility of the medical professional to make his or her own professional judgements, so as to advise and treat patients appropriately. The authors and publishers have also attempted to trace the copyright holders of all material reproduced in this publication and apologize to copyright holders if permission to publish in this form has not been obtained. If any copyright material has not been acknowledged please write and let us know so we may rectify in any future reprint.

Except as permitted under U.S. Copyright Law, no part of this book may be reprinted, reproduced, transmitted, or utilized in any form by any electronic, mechanical, or other means, now known or hereafter invented, including photocopying, microfilming, and recording, or in any information storage or retrieval system, without written permission from the publishers.

For permission to photocopy or use material electronically from this work, please access www.copyright.com (http://www.copyright.com/) or contact the Copyright Clearance Center, Inc. (CCC), 222 Rosewood Drive, Danvers, MA 01923, 978-750-8400. CCC is a not-for-profit organization that provides licenses and registration for a variety of users. For organizations that have been granted a photocopy license by the CCC, a separate system of payment has been arranged.

Trademark Notice: Product or corporate names may be trademarks or registered trademarks, and are used only for identification and explanation without intent to infringe.

Library of Congress Cataloging-in-Publication Data

Smyth, John F., author.
   Communicating with cancer patients / John F. Smyth.
   p. ; cm.
   Includes bibliographical references and index.
   ISBN 978 -1-4822-2678-2 (pbk. : alk. paper)
   I. Title.
   [DNLM: 1. Neoplasms --psychology. 2. Physician-Patient Relations. QZ 200]

RC262
616.99'40651--dc23   2013032515

Visit the Taylor & Francis Web site at
http://www.taylorandfrancis.com

and the CRC Press Web site at
http://www.crcpress.com

Dedication

For Ann, who more than anyone else has taught me
the value of good conversation.

Acknowledgement

Over the past 35 years I have been responsible for the care of more than 6000 families affected by cancer. It is they who I have to thank for teaching me the lessons that form the background of this book.

I wish to thank my colleagues and past trainees in the Edinburgh Cancer Centre for their support and collegiality. Sharing the challenges of holistic care is key to good oncology practice and I have been very fortunate to have such empathetic doctors with whom to share my own professional journey. Special thanks go to Dr Ewan Brown for his constructive comments on an earlier draft.

I wish to thank the officers of the European Society for Medical Oncology (ESMO), especially the current President, Martine Piccart, and Cora Sternberg for their encouragement to publish this book through ESMO.

A very special thank you goes to my Executive Assistant, Lisa Wood, for typing the several drafts of the manuscript and her endless patience with me in general, and my handwriting in particular!

John F Smyth

Contents

Foreword

All oncologists must be able to communicate effectively with their patients in a clear and yet sensitive way. Training in communication skills is therefore extremely important for young oncologists in preparation for the complex and often difficult conversations they will have with their patients. Although one can find various texts on the subject, this excellent book, written by Professor John Smyth, provides many insights and very useful advice drawn from his personal experiences, gained over a distinguished lifelong career as a dedicated practitioner and trainer. Young oncologists will recognise, or face, many of the situations and circumstances described by Professor Smyth, and no doubt his shared knowledge and experiences will help readers to better anticipate, prepare and communicate with their patients in the most appropriate ways possible.

Professor Smyth has held numerous important positions in the field of oncology and not least he was President of ESMO from 1991–1993 and President of the Federation of European Cancer Societies from 2005–2007. He has published extensively on a diverse range of subjects in the oncology setting and is an advisor to several governmental bodies. We are delighted and honoured to publish this book on his behalf for the benefit of ESMO's young oncologist members, as well as the wider oncology community, and thank Professor Smyth for this opportunity.

Professor Martine Piccart
ESMO President

Dr Jean-Yves Douillard
Chairman, Educational Steering Committee

Dr Lorenz Jost
Chairman, ESMO Cancer Patient Working Group

Dr Raffaele Califano
Chairman, Young Oncologist Committee

Preface

I have written this book primarily for doctors training in oncology but hopefully to be of use also for doctors in other branches of medicine and any healthcare professional involved in explaining the complexities of cancer to patients in their care. It is not a textbook but a guide, reflecting a distillation of the experience that I have gained over 30 years as a Professor of Medical Oncology, involved in the teaching of students but especially the training of young oncologists. The individual chapters address different aspects of the challenges we all face in helping anxious patients and their families to understand what is happening to them, what choices there are, and what they may expect in the months and years following a diagnosis of cancer.

Few experiences in life compare with the devastation of being told that you have cancer. Despite all the advances in our knowledge of how to manage cancer – in its many manifestations – and the real advances in survival and most particularly the *quality* of that survival, the word "cancer" still strikes fear in the minds of most people and an anticipation that life is almost over.

Information about medical advances is widely available to the public through the media and especially the internet. Curiously for the individual patient, this unselected knowledge can all too often be confusing and, far from bringing comfort, can add to their distress.

In an age of ever-increasing knowledge and its ready accessibility to the public, the role of the doctor in helping patients understand their specific circumstances has never been more important. In the days when there was little to offer, the doctor's kind words, sympathy and pastoral care were all that were expected. Nowadays patients rightfully expect their doctor to have expert knowledge, the resources to implement the best possible treatment, and the ability to explain and communicate all the complexity of this in a meaningful way. To achieve this is a very real challenge – for the doctor and the patient.

Medical students and doctors in training are faced with an enormous amount of scientific knowledge to assimilate and even experienced practitioners are challenged with keeping up to date as knowledge rapidly advances. Pre- and post-qualification, a lot of emphasis is given to teaching communication skills, and correctly so, but nothing can replace the raw experience of putting this into practice. Many medical diagnoses result in illnesses that are far worse than cancer, but given the prevailing perception in the public eye, the word "cancer" seems to have a uniquely devastating impact on people.

The "art" of cancer medicine is to develop the skills to enable you to explain what a diagnosis of cancer actually means, and the "science" surrounding the management of an individual's illness, in an intelligible and empathetic way.

The book is laid out to follow the course of conversations between physician and patient that are needed at the different stages from diagnosis to death. Following the initial shock of diagnosis, patients need to understand the reason for the various investigations required to stage their disease – an essential part of selecting optimal treatment and assigning a prognosis. In the age of multidisciplinary care, patients can easily be confused as to who is in charge of their care. Every aspect of treatment – surgery, chemotherapy, radiation treatment, often overlapping or performed simultaneously – requires explanation and understanding, and each brings the patient into contact with further teams of staff. With ever-increasing success in management, the phase of post-treatment, follow-up and monitoring (so-called "survivorship issues") presents its own difficulties for patients. Fear of relapse is very common and, if and when this happens, patients can be truly devastated. Self-confidence and faith in the medical profession can be lost; you have to try to restore both. Patients may then face further treatment and in many cases eventually progression to the terminal phase of their illness.

I have written a short chapter on research. Progress can only result from research. Encouraging patient participation through explaining the reasoning behind a research study and the various responsibilities involved for both the doctor and the patient is a vital part of modern cancer care. However, the common theme throughout all these pages emphasises your prime responsibility to create confidence and reassurance for your patient. Introducing the concept of research inevitably questions current knowledge, introduces uncertain choice and, if not well explained, can undermine the impression that you have the knowledge and resources to offer the best possible care. Explaining research can be really challenging.

The final chapter discusses a few aspects of complementary and alternative medicine (CAM). I deliberately left this till last in order to encompass conversations that are almost inevitable with every patient that you will meet. However, CAM is increasingly being used and the concept of "integrative oncology" seeks to embrace CAM within conventional medicine. CAM is complex – physically and psychologically. Prescribers and patients sometimes have an evidence base on which to rely, but sometimes "belief" is sufficient. There are benefits and pitfalls and I allude to some of both of these. At each and every stage of this so-called "journey", the patient needs help to understand and, at whatever level possible, come to terms with what is happening. The interaction between doctor, patient and their family is critical and varies at the different stages of an individual's illness. I have separated these various stages into separate chapters, but of course there is continuity to the whole experience.

The advice offered is written in the form of conversations between me and a trainee oncologist. A given knowledge of general medicine is therefore assumed and the emphasis is very much on the "art of medicine" and how to practice it, rather than the "science", which is more readily taught and learned. The traditions of British medical education and training used to be based on an apprenticeship model: students learned from young doctors, and doctors in training learned from their seniors and particularly consultants or specialists. In my own experience, the benefit of being allowed to "sit in" on specialist consultations to observe the conduct of and, most particularly, the mode of conversation between skilled communicators and their patients was both a privilege and an excellent foundation for developing my own personal approach. The classic ward round where a consultant would be accompanied by trainee doctors and nurses going from bed to bed in a hushed ward where there were no visitors or other extraneous diversions may have had an element of theatre, but the opportunity to observe and listen to the conversations and method of explanation in this setting was a very important part of training in this difficult area of medicine. Hospital-based clinical practice has changed and for a variety of reasons there are many fewer opportunities nowadays for trainee doctors to "sit in" and observe their seniors or to accompany them on the wards in the way that I have described. It is not only the older generation of doctors who regret this loss of apprenticeship in favour of much greater emphasis on doctors becoming self-taught. I hope that my reflections in these pages do not appear patronising or prescriptive. Where the "art of medicine" is concerned, every doctor must develop their own style of communication. What is offered here is intended to help trainees to develop and hone their own skills in this most challenging but rewarding practice of medicine.

Chapter 1 Introduction

This book describes ways to converse with cancer patients in order to help them understand the nature of their illness and the complex management thereof. Conversation involves talking *and* listening. In this regard, your primary responsibility as a doctor is to explain the medical facts about a patient's illness and to advise on management. With practice this is not difficult to accomplish – "listening" is much harder, but is absolutely essential. The overriding emotion surrounding conversations about cancer is that of anxiety. Patients are afraid – afraid of the whole concept of a life-threatening disease, afraid of its treatment and afraid that they are going to die sooner than they had expected. In professional life, your time with an individual patient will always be limited and there is much that you have to say in explaining the complexity of cancer. However, it is vital to allow time for the patient to express their own personal concerns to enable you to focus on the particular aspects that are of immediate relevance to them at this time.

One of your principal responsibilities is to create the appropriate balance between hope and truthfulness. Hopelessness is an overwhelmingly distressing emotion that can obliterate any positive aspect concerning the quality of a patient's life. There are occasional situations in oncology practice that are truly hopeless – but these are rare. With modern medical management it is possible to help virtually everyone – to a greater or lesser extent. Therefore without minimising the seriousness of the situation, you should try to explain that there are known pathways of treatment, that their circumstances are not unique, and that you can propose plans to give patients a way to look forward. Helping them to realise that they are not alone, but that you have a team of professionals to care for them, can be of inestimable value at the time of diagnosis. Relieving any initial sense of complete hopelessness, right from the very first consultation, can be of enormous benefit to patients and their families. It is, however, essential that you avoid being inappropriately positive, thereby raising false hope. You must try to strike the right balance between telling the truth, but leaving some positive element of hope – where this is appropriate, as it usually is. This is achieved by explaining the evidence on which we base our management decisions.

So talking and listening are key skills that must be fine-tuned by everyone involved in cancer management. In the following pages I offer some advice about the necessary content of key conversations and the styles of language that may be used. Different phases of treatment require different approaches. We anticipate different goals which are appropriate to the initial phase of coming to terms with the diagnosis, through the active phases of treatment and follow-up, to eventual progression.

Right from the beginning it is important to establish with a patient the terminology that you will use in all your conversations. Some patients are comfortable to use the word "cancer"; others may prefer to use the word "tumour" or "malignancy" or "growth", or even "my illness". The choice of specific term is not important, but it is helpful to establish the language that you will subsequently use – to avoid confusion or, more probably, assumed confusion, which is part of a denial process. The word "cancer" encompasses a large number of different forms of malignancy and there is a wide spectrum of illness involved. Of course the symptoms, signs and prognosis of chronic lymphocytic leukaemia are totally different from those of pancreatic or breast cancer. The former may be detected without symptoms, may not require immediate intervention and may be compatible with life expectancy measured in several years. A patient with pancreatic cancer may give a history of rapid transition from good health to illness with major symptoms of anorexia, weight loss and pain, and have a life expectancy of only a few months. For newly diagnosed patients with breast cancer, there are issues of sexuality, complex prolonged multi-modal therapy and an uncertain life expectancy. What is most important to appreciate is that patients will be referred to you from very different starting points. The heavy smoker who has been coughing up blood and losing weight is not going to be too surprised when he has to be told that he has lung cancer. The patient who has all the signs and symptoms of profound cachexia may very well suspect cancer when their pancreatic tumour causes frank jaundice. However, the vague symptoms of anaemia and fatigue that may be the prelude to a chronic leukaemia or myeloma may not awaken fears of malignancy, and the diagnosis comes as a much greater shock. Breast cancer can be particularly brutal since patients are often well and asymptomatic until suddenly finding a lump in their breast or axilla. The oncologist requires not only an understanding of the presentation and management of this variety of disease, but most importantly an alertness and ability to adapt their communications to the different situations that individual patients require.

On being diagnosed with cancer, patients often ask : "Why me?" and, aside from seeking answers about genetic predisposition, family risk, or the guilt-provoking lifestyle factors such as tobacco, alcohol, obesity, etc., they need a brief explanation of the biology of cancer – what is a tumour? – and especially the significance of metastases. Suggested ways to explain this are dealt with later, but an early explanation of these processes will help a new patient to understand the need for staging their illness and, where appropriate, the complexity of multi-modal treatment.

The different phases of management

As soon as possible after being told of their diagnosis, patients should be given an outline of the different phases of management, as illustrated in Figure 1.

Figure 1: Tumour growth during different phases of disease management.

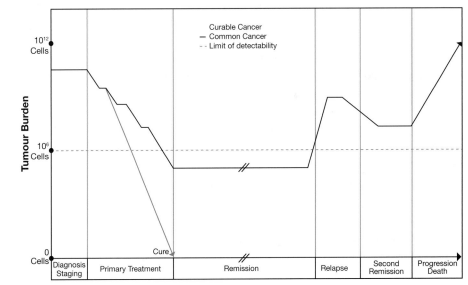

Each of these phases is the subject of a separate chapter and requires different levels of communication. Nowadays there are rare situations where, because of extreme old age, frailty or comorbid disease or the extent of disease at presentation, it is inappropriate to investigate further or consider active anti-cancer treatment. However, for the great majority of newly diagnosed patients it is reassuring to outline the phase of initial investigations, the detailed pathology and staging followed by treatment, the variable outcomes of this and therefore the need for follow-up. In introducing the concept that further treatment may potentially be needed in due course, the concept of control as opposed to cure can be introduced and, for patients who wish it, a discussion of life expectancy and death. Advice on how to approach these different aspects of management is discussed in the subsequent chapters.

The X axis of Figure 1 represents time – from diagnosis to death. After diagnosis, investigations are made to assess the presence and extent of tumour invasion and spread (metastases) in order to select appropriate treatment and to inform the prognosis – equally as important to the doctor as to the patient. On the Y axis is tumour burden, here presented by cell number. It is estimated that a tumour burden of greater than 10^{12} cells is incompatible with life. To reach a size sufficient to cause symptoms, many tumours consist of more than 10^{10} cells. Following the period of initial treatment – surgery, radiation, hormone treatment, medicines or a combination of these – a successfully treated tumour will have shrunk to 10^6 cells or less. Since a tumour size of one cubic centimetre will contain about 10^8 cells, it is not surprising that 10^6 cells is below the level of detectability either clinically or with conventional radiological means. What we choose to call a "complete response" may, in the rare cases where such is possible, represent total eradication of the tumour, i.e. cure – for example, achievable in testis cancer. All too often, however, complete remission simply reflects the absence of our ability to detect small volume disease. With the increasing use of biomarkers and developments in imaging, this limit of detectability is going down. The difference between cure and recurrent disease is of course a reflection of the survival of some malignant cells following initial treatment, re-emerging over time as a "recurrence" or "relapse". The interval between the end of initial treatment and recurrence – so-called "remission" – requires monitoring by the doctor and patient. Good communication is an essential factor in helping patients develop the optimal quality of their lives during this period before the devastation of a relapse. Where appropriate, second- and third-line treatment may be given to provide a possible second, usually partial, remission before eventual tumour progression and death.

Figure 2: Fluctuating levels of anxiety at different phases of disease management.

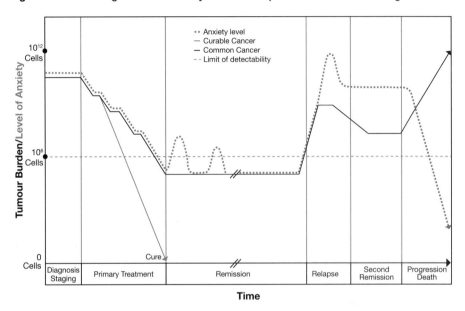

Figure 2 shows the same graph of tumour burden over time as Figure 1, but with a diagram of patient anxiety superimposed. High levels of anxiety are to be expected at diagnosis but, with effective treatment and good communication, patients should be helped greatly to reduce this anxiety by the time initial treatment is completed. As discussed in Chapter 5, remission can be associated with episodes of renewed anxiety, but the moment of relapse is often associated with levels of anxiety and depression that exceed even those experienced at diagnosis. With good palliative care, the period leading up to death should be accompanied by a resolution of anxiety and its replacement with a sense of calm and peace.

Especially for non-oncologists using this book, it may be helpful to outline the basics of what we currently know about the aetiology of a tumour that brings a patient to your care. In my experience, patients find it hard to accept that the process may have been going on in their bodies for a long time, such that the presentation of a tumour is in fact biologically a late effect. Depending on many individual factors, not least their scientific and medical knowledge, or lack of it, different patients will seek different levels of explanation about what has led up to their diagnosis. Recognising this variability, the oncologist should be prepared to give an appropriate précis of the essential basic facts.

The aetiology of cancer

In the Western world, one in three people now develop cancer. The statistics for incidence and survival vary considerably in different parts of the world. This book is not the place to discuss such variation, but factors that influence this include the accuracy and completeness of data collection and, naturally, access to the best possible treatment. Such facts and figures are important in planning healthcare on a population basis, but the individual patient is concerned only with factors that may have been responsible for their own specific illness. We now believe that cancer is caused by a mixture of "seed and soil". In this terminology, the seed represents known or unknown carcinogens, such as tobacco, alcohol, excess sunlight and carcinogens in our food, or spontaneous mutations; the soil represents our individual genetic makeup that renders us either more or less susceptible to the tumour-promoting seed that interacts with that genetic background.

I have found it useful to help patients understand that cancer is a natural phenomenon. I try to explain that our bodies cannot develop, grow and maintain themselves without cell division and, like every other natural phenomenon, the process of cell division does not happen in a one hundred per cent perfect way. The number of cells dividing in an adult's body within each 24-hour period is phenomenal. One example of this is that in our bone marrow, in each 24-hour period, we produce over 70 billion neutrophils and 200 billion red cells. Quite an opportunity for mistakes to happen! With advancing age, repair and renewal systems break down, mistakes occur, cell division can go wrong and even one such error can result in uncontrolled cell replication leading to malignant growth – i.e. a cancer. Whether the damage to genetic DNA occurs spontaneously or in response to environmental carcinogens, repair mechanisms have evolved to remove or repair damaged DNA which could otherwise cause unregulated cell division leading to tumour development. We have also evolved other "housekeeping" mechanisms known as tumour suppressor genes, whose function is to suppress the process of faulty, potentially oncogenic, cell division. Faults in the machinery of tumour suppression and DNA repair can be inherited, and this explains the basis of some forms of familial or inherited cancer.

Many patients will ask you about genetic risk and cancer. They are curious to know if they themselves inherited a cancer risk, but usually are more concerned for their siblings and children. As our knowledge of familial cancer increases, so does the complexity of explanation – and, most importantly, the need for detailed interrogation of a patient's true genetic history. Breast cancer is a good example.

It is now thought that 5–10% of all breast cancers are due to inheritance of high-penetrance genes transmitted in an autosomal dominant fashion. Pathogenic mutations in the gene known as *BRCA1* confer a lifetime risk of breast cancer of between 80–85%. Normal *BRCA1* produces a protein required for DNA repair and the regulation of cell-cycle progression. A related gene, *BRCA2*, is similarly involved in repair processes and, together, mutations in these genes account for about 20% of familial breast cancer. It is now possible to screen women for mutations in these genes, which is relevant not only to the individual, but may also be relevant to daughters and other family members; this is referred to again in Chapter 2.

Apart from the need to interrogate a patient's genetic history accurately, the explanation of inherited risk and its implications is complex and time consuming. Wherever possible, if you suspect a familial contribution, it is best to refer the patient to a genetic counselling service, which has the expertise and time to investigate this further. This is referred to again in Chapter 2.

With our current level of knowledge, we believe that inherited susceptibility is rare and often expressed as cancers presenting at a relatively early age, but the more common acquired faults – resulting from the loss of "housekeeping" – explain why cancers mostly develop with advanced age: the sixth, seventh and eighth decades of life. By the age of 70, a human being has had more than 25,500 days for things to go wrong – and they do. The machinery wears out and the malignant cell division escapes to form a cancer. Whilst describing cancer as part of a "natural phenomenon", it must be appreciated that the development of a tumour is biologically a very rare event. However, the similarity of cancer cell division to the process of normal cell division partly explains why it is so very difficult to design anti-cancer therapies that destroy abnormal growth without irreparably harming normal growth in host tissues.

In trying to explain to patients why it is so difficult to design an anti-cancer drug, I often use the example of antibiotics. The latter can be designed to interfere with the metabolism of a bacterium whose chemistry is sufficiently different to that of a mammalian cell to allow specificity. The bacterium is killed, the host is not. By contrast, to design a molecule that can destroy a breast cancer cell or a malignant lymphocyte, without causing irreparable harm to the neighbouring normal breast cells or lymphocytes, is a very real challenge. There *are* real differences in the metabolism of a cancer cell to that of the normal counterpart, but the differences are often quantitative, not qualitative – hence the narrow therapeutic index of so many anti-cancer drugs.

As our knowledge of familial cancer and the effects of the environment on the causes of sporadic cancers improve, we increasingly hope to develop new strategies for the prevention of cancer. This knowledge also informs screening techniques to detect tumours before they cause clinical illness. It is essential for the specialist oncologist to be aware of these developments, since patients may well need help in coming to terms with their diagnosis, if they have been previously tested for familial cancer but develop a spontaneous one, or more commonly have been attending screening clinics but develop a so-called "interval" cancer in between.

Let us now consider the beginning of the patient's experience of cancer: diagnosis and staging.

Chapter 2 **Diagnosis and Staging**

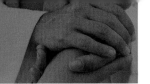

As a trainee oncologist, one of your most daunting responsibilities is to learn how to conduct a new patient "interview". For the newly diagnosed patient, it is impossible to exaggerate the importance of the first consultation with a specialist oncologist. You are unlikely to be the first person to tell the patient that they have cancer, but you are the key person in whom trust will be placed to know what to do to achieve the best possible outcome.

Oncologists rarely diagnose cancer – usually patients are referred to them after initial diagnosis by others (see below), but your conduct of the first "specialist" appointment is critical to a patient's understanding of what is happening to them, their coming to terms with this and helping them to understand what they can expect in the near future and beyond. With time and experience you will derive a sense of achievement when you conduct these first consultations well, but it is a real challenge, especially when you are learning how to do this. Many factors contribute to make this initial conversation difficult, but let us first consider the "ideal situation" where you perform well, the environment helps you and the patient is reassured. In the box below are listed the ten elements that you must try to address during the first consultation. Not all of these factors are in your control. One of the most important issues is how long you have available for the first consultation. Too short a time is insulting and frustrating for both you and the patient. Conversely, if you take too long by going into too much detail, you may miss the primary objective, i.e. to assess the history and findings on examination, and formulate a management plan that may take you to further investigations (staging) or may directly involve treatment. This objective must be accomplished in a prescribed time (always too short) whilst generating a sense of confidence and relieving anxiety. It is a challenge. Let us dissect the process into its various components.

1. Environment

2. Referral letter

3. Results and investigations to date

4. Observation

5. History

1. Environment

New patients are usually seen in the privacy of the outpatient setting, but you may meet them on a busy hospital ward, and it may or may not be possible for you to influence the ambience in which you see patients for the first time. Inevitably many hospital clinics are noisy and frenetic. Most particularly for this first appointment, a peaceful setting is ideally preferred, i.e. one where there is not too much environmental noise, not too many patients or staff rushing around, no building works taking place immediately next to you and, if you are fortunate, no mobile phones or pagers going off during your consultation. Experienced doctors will recognise all of the above, but some of these factors are in fact within your control, such as leaving mobile phones outside the consulting room – especially for first consultations.

2. Referral letter

Since most patients present with the symptoms of cancer to doctors who are not cancer specialists, it is usual for patients to be referred to you who are already informed of their diagnosis. A good referral letter will help you to estimate what the patient may or may not know at the time of first meeting you as the specialist. The difference between receiving a well-written and thorough referral letter compared with a short account of an operation or a tissue diagnosis can make an enormous difference to your conduct of the first consultation.

Ideally a referral letter should explain not only the presentation of the symptoms and signs that led to the diagnosis, but how the latter was established and most particularly what the patient has been told. A good referral letter will also tell you something of the past medical history and the social setting of the patient in terms of occupation, marital status, family, etc. It is to be hoped that, before long, all medical records will be kept electronically in a way that will allow you to access all previous medical experience, and the results and investigations of relevance to the current problem, prior to meeting the patient for the first time. Where your practice involves regular referrals from known colleagues, it is possible over time to teach them the inestimable value of a thorough referral letter. Patients may justifiably expect you to be fully aware of their relevant previous medical history, the presenting symptoms of this illness, investigations to date, etc. etc., and when you can demonstrate knowledge of this it is greatly reassuring to the patient that there is continuity of care in their referral. However, such information is not always made available and suggestions for how you deal with this are referred to below.

3. Results and investigations to date

From the referral letter it is important to establish what investigations have been carried out to date and the results of these. Patients will be very surprised and disappointed if a series of radiological investigations or blood tests have already been performed and yet you as the specialist are not yet aware of the results. I strongly advise you to take the time to read the referral letter carefully and any accompanying medical records as thoroughly as possible, before you call the patient into your consulting room. At all costs you should avoid sitting a patient next to you and then starting to read their history – you can of course refer back to such a referral letter or other medical notes for points of detail, but the more that you know about the patient before you first meet them, the greater will be their confidence in you and the department in which they are to be looked after.

4. Observation

A great deal can be learned about a patient's state of mind and attitude to their recent diagnosis purely by observing them. For many years I had the luxury of a consulting room that was the furthest walking distance from the waiting area. By observing patients walking even a short distance, you can gain invaluable information about their appearance, their ease of movement and their mood – all of which inform you about elements of their physical and mental health which contribute to your assessment of their overall health and what we call their "performance status". As a patient enters your consulting room, it is of course essential to introduce yourself and, by shaking hands, you establish an important physical contact with your patient which can be significantly reassuring for them. This introduction also applies to anyone accompanying your patient: a partner, husband, wife, close relative or friend. As you invite the patient to sit, you will notice their physical deportment and aspects of their physical wellbeing that are immediately observable – the state of their hair, skin, hands and clothing – all of which give useful clues to inform you about the level of distress that the patient has already experienced.

Observation of the patient's hands provides a particular opportunity to gather information about their state of mind – the difference between well-manicured or neglected finger nails, and whether the patient is able to relax or constantly fidgets with their hands, are all important clues to their mental state. As an oncologist, you appreciate the overwhelming importance of anxiety. When teaching medical students in the oncology clinic, I remind them that every single patient in the waiting area and most of their accompanying friends and relatives have a very high level of anxiety, most especially those awaiting their first consultation. Probably the most important aspect of the new patient consultation where you can give immediate help to the patient is to reduce that level of anxiety and help them find some reassurance in what you are able to explain to them.

5. History

Unless you are fortunate to have an extremely comprehensive referral letter, in almost all cases during a first consultation you will want to take a history of the patient's illness for yourself. Depending of course on the level of detail in the referral letter, I recommend that you start your conversation with something like, "Can you tell me what you have understood about the reasons for being referred to me today?" By opening your conversation with such a statement, you invite the patient to immediately share with you their level of knowledge of their current health and the experience they have had since being told their diagnosis. It is for you to assess what they may have *actually* been told versus what they have *understood*, and the same applies to any accompanying relative or close friend.

Discrepancies between what has actually been said to patients and what they have comprehended are very well documented. Sometimes the blame lies with us in the medical profession for using the wrong language or for giving too much or too little detail, but very often what is reported back to you is the result of sifting information that the patient either has not understood or does not wish to address, whilst retaining more hopeful positive elements of what they have been told. In some situations the shock of diagnosis alone renders them unable to register and recall any further information. In establishing what the patient knows of their existing condition, you may be faced with a barrage of questions about "What did Doctor X mean by …?" or what is the consequence of a specific symptom or sign that has been explained? My advice to you is to store any response to such questions at this stage of the consultation, and allow yourself time to rehearse your own plan of action before explaining what the next steps will be. You can then answer collectively questions that have arisen both before and during this first consultation. You might therefore say, "May I answer that in a moment, when I have asked you a few more questions of my own". If you have been given inadequate or very little information about the symptoms and signs leading to the diagnosis, I would recommend that you start your own history-taking with sentences such as, "Allow me just to go back over the start of your illness, the way it all presented".

After these preliminaries, you hopefully will have established some reassurance in the patient's mind that you understand what has happened to them in the past and particularly that you have elicited and taken account of their *specific* concerns. You can then proceed to take a conventional history. This should cover the past as well as the current illness. Obtaining a history of past medical problems is important for two reasons. Firstly, prior illness may have affected, or continue to influence, present health, especially a chronic illness such as cardiac, respiratory or renal problems, diabetes, arthritis, etc. Impaired organ function may be relevant to your choice of anti-cancer medicines, and of course it is essential to document carefully any current medication that the patient is taking, not least to be aware of potential drug interactions when prescribing multiple anti-cancer drugs.

The second reason that it is important to discuss past medical problems is that it allows you to assess the attitude of your patient to doctors, nurses, hospitals, etc. If previous medical interventions have been positive, it may help to lessen the anxiety associated with the new diagnosis of cancer. If, however, past experiences have been less favourable, anxiety may be heightened, and it is important to try to separate those experiences from this new episode of serious ill health. An important part of the history-taking should involve information about lifestyle factors – the consumption of tobacco and alcohol are obvious ones – and any peculiarities in diet that might be relevant to management.

Family history is important, as discussed below. Other health issues include concurrent medication and of course the symptoms of this particular illness. In taking a social history, occupation can be particularly important. This may lead you to clues as to the patient's concern that such a serious diagnosis as cancer may curtail their ambitions in their work environment. This can significantly add to the depressing reality of their diagnosis. Conversely there are patients for whom the diagnosis of cancer allows them to take early retirement from work that they disliked, and to concentrate on social and family aspects of their lives that have been neglected for far too long. In documenting their marital status and the age and stage of children, you will similarly be given clues, sometimes very bluntly, about thwarted ambition – the desire to have children, the desire to see children grow up, anticipated grandchildren, etc. At this stage in the first consultation, you may well have to be prepared for significant emotional responses, tearfulness and an inability to continue the conversation. Patients are frequently embarrassed by such totally natural and understandable reactions and you should reassure them that such behaviour is neither a surprise nor an embarrassment to you. It is not only psychiatrists who understand the value of silence and sometimes it is better that you simply refer back to reading medical notes or to your own annotations whilst giving the patient time to compose themselves.

Family history is important for two reasons. Firstly, you need to know about dependent children or adults and the relevant demands that they may place on your patient. Secondly, it may be appropriate to know about the possibility of inherited cancer – both for your patient's management but also in case it is relevant to screen other family members. Our understanding of the genetics of cancer is developing rapidly and details of current knowledge are beyond the scope of this book, but the example of breast cancer may serve to warn you of the type of question that may be posed to you and of your need to keep abreast of this developing field. As mentioned briefly in Chapter 1, it is now possible to screen women with breast cancer for mutations in *BRCA1* and *BRCA2* genes. Where this is indicated, it is important to establish the presence or absence of these mutations, since they can have a direct bearing on the management of the breast cancer, but also unfortunately these mutations also carry an increased risk of ovarian and other cancers.

The starting point for establishing whether or not the patient has an inherited cancer is to take a detailed family history. It may not be appropriate for you to attempt this during the first consultation, but where suspicion is high (for example, if there are several siblings and/or a parent with the same disease) it is preferable to refer patients to a genetic clinic where detailed pedigrees can be established. In the UK there are now published guidelines to categorise women into low, medium and high risk of inherited breast cancer. Women at medium risk can be assessed and managed at secondary level, i.e. a hospital-based oncology centre, and only those at high risk should be referred to the regional genetics service. Your major responsibility is to know the criteria for assigning risk so that you can refer appropriately.

The aim of taking your own history is not only to establish the basic medical facts upon which you will base decisions about treatment options and prognosis, but also to get a first feeling for the emotional environment in which your patient exists. Anxiety bordering on fear of an imminent death is not unusual amongst patients of all educational backgrounds, and one of the ways in which you can help patients during the course of their early treatment, before you know to what level they will benefit from this, is to understand as much as you can glean about the social, environmental and support structures that are available for your patient. I could easily fill this book with anecdotes of particular situations, but maybe two will suffice. The first is the importance of pet animals in addition to human family members.

I well remember an elderly gentleman diagnosed with advanced melanoma, a condition for which there were, at the time, few options for influencing life expectancy. Having worked as a forester all his life, he attended his first outpatient appointment with his daughter, a qualified nurse. The patient lived in a humble cottage by the sea, which he shared with an elderly dog, of which he was clearly extremely fond. The daughter wished him to leave the cottage and live with her when they were informed that his life expectancy was probably only a few months. The patient politely refused this offer but needed my help to support him in explaining this to his loving daughter. He wished to live his short remaining time able to sit outside his cottage watching the sun set with his elderly dog – there being no room for the latter in his daughter's house. The daughter needed help in accepting that the dog's care was both more useful and important than medical interventions or even her daughterly love, which had to be expressed in other ways. Three months later she returned to my clinic to inform me of her father's peaceful death and that the dog had outlived him by only a few days – unquestionably the patient was right! It is not for us as doctors to referee between family members, but sometimes you can steer decisions in a useful way, respecting always that the wishes of your patient should come first.

Another anecdote which is worth reporting relates to the problem that you will all encounter sooner or later – that of a poor referral letter for a patient who you are meeting for the first time. I well remember calling out the name of a male patient in the waiting area and seeing a man in his late sixties stand up and approach me. He was dressed in an expensive but faded sweater and corduroy trousers with shoes that had not seen polish for some while. The referral letter gave me significant detail about a melanoma that had been resected recently from his left shoulder, but told me nothing else whatsoever about him, apart from his date of birth. Knowing so little about him, I decided to be completely honest and explained that despite the fact that he had been through the surgical department in my own hospital, I knew a great deal about his left shoulder but absolutely nothing about him. Embarrassing as that was both for me and the hospital administration, I felt it best to start from the beginning. His silence and stern face confirmed my suspicions that he had already lost total confidence in me and our hospital. Nevertheless I said directly to him, "Can you please tell me what you do for an occupation?" His reply was, "You will be glad that you asked because I am a Senior Law Lord (Judge) and I specialise in medical negligence!" Probably easier that I was a professor than a trainee at the time, but my experience told me just to take a deep breath and keep looking straight at the patient. A broad grin slowly broke on his face, the ice was broken, he thanked me for my common sense, some confidence was restored and over the next three years we became firm friends.

6. Examination

An essential part of your first consultation is to examine the patient thoroughly. This offers an opportunity to develop further your knowledge of the patient's lifestyle and, whilst the patient is undressing, to address questions to the accompanying partner or friend. Only do this within the listening capacity of the patient. The days of informing a husband about his wife's illness without the wife knowing first, or vice versa, are fortunately long gone. Having completed your examination, and whilst the patient is dressing, you have a brief time to think. My advice is that you should actually say that you wish to do so. Whilst making your own notes, if appropriate you can look back through referral letters or notes and take the time to gather your thoughts. Rather than using inappropriate social conversation whilst a patient is dressing, it is far better to have time to reflect on what you are going to say and do next.

7. Performance status

By the time that you have completed your history and examination, you are able to decide on what we call the patient's "performance status (PS)". Ever since the pioneering days of Dr David Karnofsky in the late 1940s, we have appreciated the enormous importance of a patient's global health in relationship to prognosis in general, and ability to cope with differing intensities of treatment in particular. Several scales of PS are in use, including the original Karnofsky scale based on a percentage allocation and the Eastern Cooperative Oncology Group (ECOG) scale, as illustrated in the following tables.

Karnofsky Scale

- 100% – normal, no complaints, no signs of disease.
- 90% – capable of normal activity, few symptoms or signs of disease.
- 80% – normal activity with some difficulty, some symptoms or signs.
- 70% – caring for self, not capable of normal activity or work.
- 60% – requiring some help, can take care of most personal requirements.
- 50% – requires help often, requires frequent medical care.
- 40% – disabled, requires special care and help.
- 30% – severely disabled, hospital admission indicated but no risk of death.
- 20% – very ill, urgently requiring admission, requires supportive measures or treatment.
- 10% – moribund, rapidly progressive fatal disease processes.
- 0% – death.

ECOG Scale

0	Asymptomatic	Fully active, able to carry on all predisease activities without restriction.
1	Symptomatic but completely ambulatory	Restricted in physically strenuous activity but ambulatory and able to carry out work of a light or sedentary nature. For example, light housework, office work.
2	Symptomatic, <50% in bed during the day	Ambulatory and capable of all self-care but unable to carry out any work activities. Up and about more than 50% of waking hours.
3	Symptomatic, >50% in bed, but not bedbound	Capable of only limited self-care, confined to bed or chair 50% or more of waking hours
4	Bedbound	Completely disabled. Cannot carry on any self-care. Totally confined to bed or chair.
5	Death	

With experience it is not difficult to assign a PS to any given patient on any given day – but it is important to appreciate that PS can and does change over the course of ill health. Severe symptoms and signs of diagnosis may lead to a poor PS, but if management is effective the PS should improve over time. Deciding on a patient's PS at diagnosis may have a major role in your decision about initial treatment: highly challenging (toxic) treatment is poorly tolerated by patients with a poor PS and therefore contraindicated, but you do not want to under-treat patients where PS is good. If initially poor PS improves, you can reconsider the level of treatment being recommended, and similarly, if disease fails to respond or progresses after initial success, a decreasing PS should influence your recommendation to reduce or even stop active treatment.

8. Investigations

For the majority of new patient referrals, some preliminary investigations will already have been performed, but you will almost certainly want to carry out further staging investigations. Despite the pressure on time during a first consultation, it is essential that you explain the reasoning for doing staging investigations – this is often overlooked. Simply explaining that it is standard practice to perform certain radiological or haematological investigations is not sufficient. A patient with a newly diagnosed lump in the breast will not automatically understand why you want to investigate their bones or scan their liver. A patient presenting with a melanoma on their leg may be extremely frightened by the thought of a brain scan to exclude metastases unless you use the right language to explain the reasons for this procedure.

Most patients are aware of the concept of metastasis and the life-threatening potential that this represents. When describing the need to investigate for this, I use phrases such as, "In order to choose the most appropriate treatment, we routinely look to see if there is any evidence of secondary spread". (If the topic has come up in earlier conversation, I refer back to the concept that cancer does not arise suddenly but may have been present in a silent form for some considerable time.) Depending on the disease in question, you then go on to explain that breast or prostate cancer often spreads to bone, that colorectal cancer often spreads to the liver, etc. You must be prepared for some patients to be considerably surprised by this, most particularly if there are no symptoms to suggest that metastases may be present. Particularly in the case of clinical trial protocols, patients often feel overwhelmed by the number of investigations recommended. In this situation it may be possible to divide the workload of explaining this between yourself and a clinical nurse specialist (see Chapter 4), who can elaborate further on the need for doing particular investigations, since this avoids overload of information during the first consultation. The important point is to make sure that the patient understands the reason for needing to look beyond the obvious site of origin of their cancer.

9. Next steps

The penultimate stage of the initial consultation should be to explain what will happen to the patient next. This will probably be undergoing the further staging investigations referred to above. You will judge the time taken to complete those and therefore when to see the patient for the second time. If the treatment plan is obvious and is to be started in the near future, it is naturally important to outline the treatment involved; this is discussed in the next chapter. The most important aspect of explaining the next steps is to give the patient the reassurance that they are now part of a system that will look after them, and help them come to terms with their diagnosis and understand what is happening to them. Giving patients a plan or framework of what will happen over the forthcoming weeks and months is very reassuring at a time when their emotions are running high, and their anxiety is making it difficult for them to comprehend not only what is happening to them, but also what is being explained. Creating a structure that is personalised to their needs can help greatly to reassure patients that not everything in their lives has come unstuck at the same time.

10. Questions

Having completed your part of the explanation, it is important to give the patient and accompanying people an opportunity to ask questions. In some instances, patients may be so exhausted by the emotional experience they have just been through that they seem surprisingly uninterested in asking further questions at this time. Other patients will have too many questions for the time that you have allocated. In my experience, patients will often confront you right at the beginning of their whole experience of cancer with questions about mortality: "Am I dying and how long have I got?" I refer to questions about death in Chapter 6, but my advice is not to avoid discussion about mortality even at a first consultation. Any attempt to cheer patients up and dismiss the ultimate consequence of cancer is condescending and creates a distance between you and the patient, which is exactly the opposite of what you wish to establish. With the exception of the very elderly patient whose illness may be so advanced that death is obviously imminent, I recommend that you do not assign figures of life expectancy to patients during a first consultation. In truth, at an early stage of investigation and treatment planning, you may be unable to give an accurate prognosis with many cancers, particularly concerning life expectancy. Even with cancers such as pancreatic cancer, which all too often are associated with a very short life expectancy, it may be reasonable to explain that survival may be measured in months rather than years, but I would advise against being more specific at this early stage.

When challenged directly by the question, "How long have I got?", I have often replied, "I honestly do not know. I am not trying to avoid giving you an answer, but your outlook depends on many things – not least your response to the treatment that we are proposing. Some patients derive considerable benefit, others less so. We have to wait and see, but your prognosis will become much clearer in a few weeks' time." This type of language avoids a brutal, nihilistic statement, avoids a commitment which in all truth you cannot be certain of, and allows the patient an appropriate sense of hope that can be reassuring, not misleading. The important thing is not to avoid the question, but to leave the answer open by explaining that this will depend on the results of investigations, the treatment plan to be established when those investigations have been completed, and most importantly the patient's response or otherwise to treatment.

Patients often ask for advice as to whether to continue at work or to retire; my advice in that situation is to temporise for the same reasons as mentioned above with prognosis. Decisions made too hastily are often the wrong ones and, although there are exceptions, most employers are sympathetic to these circumstances and even the self-employed have some window of time to decide what they wish to do when confronted with serious illness. Another anecdote that will always remain with me is of a man in his late middle age, newly diagnosed with carcinoma of the colon which, with the combination of surgery and chemotherapy, had a reasonable prognosis. This bachelor, who had never had any ill health in his life, returned for his second appointment to inform me that having cancer, assuming he only had a short time to live, he had resigned from his job, sold his house and had his dog destroyed. At a follow-up appointment some three years later, he recounted how utterly distressed he was that he had made such poor decisions in a hurry and against medical advice.

Similarly for carers, there may be difficult decisions to be addressed with regard to work: "Should I retire now to look after my wife/husband?" "What will happen if they die and I have given up my income too soon?" etc. etc. Families should be advised to take their time with such emotionally challenging dilemmas.

As an oncologist dealing with serious illness and a highly anxious new patient, you must be prepared for the unexpected questions which are designed more to probe your openness about prognosis than the question might obviously deserve. Women of childbearing age may well ask whether you think it is wise for them to continue planning to have further children – they are simply asking whether they are going to be alive in 5–10 years or 5–10 months.

Whilst greatly welcoming and encouraging new patients to present with their closest member of family or friend, both for support but also to help them interpret what has been explained to them, where possible I do discourage younger patients from arriving at a new patient interview with small children. The distraction of having to entertain small children whilst undergoing such an important conversation is obvious, but another anecdote may be illustrative. A highly intelligent woman in her late thirties presented as a new patient with metastatic breast cancer. In addition to two older children she had a two-year-old, who she brought not only to her first consultation, but to every subsequent appointment. The child disliked hospitals, disliked white coats and inevitably therefore, I am sorry to say, probably disliked me! It was obvious that there were others who could have looked after the daughter for the short period of time required, but the child's presence was a very clear aggressive statement to me and other medical staff that the patient was determined to live to see this little girl grow up, and we should never be allowed to forget that.

Patients with young children (5–15 years or so) have very particular challenges. Apart from the obvious anxiety about whether or not they will survive to see their children grow up, there is the immediate problem of what to say to them about having cancer. I have often been asked for advice about this. Any advice that you offer will naturally have to take into account the specific circumstances of the family concerned – the patient's probable prognosis, the degree of educational understanding of both parent and children, the age of the children, etc. Some patients choose to keep their illness a secret from their children – and these patients may never ask for your opinion – but as a general rule I encourage parents to be as open and honest with their children as they feel comfortable so to do. They do not have to explain the situation in any great detail, but I advise them at least to explain to their children that they have cancer, that they will have to attend the hospital or clinic for treatment and follow-up, and, where relevant, to give warning in advance of any obvious physical side effects such as hair loss or other changes in appearance. In my experience, children are remarkably accepting of this type of information, even if their comprehension is limited. The risk of avoiding any discussion, or worse of inventing false alibis for hospital visits, is that children are so often more aware of life around them than we give them credit for. Children talk to other children, both at home and at school, and if a child suspects or works out for themselves that their parent has a serious medical problem that is being kept from them, they may well jump to a conclusion that is far worse than the reality of the situation – "Mummy must be about to die", etc. This can cause far more distress than an appropriate sharing of what is indeed a serious problem affecting the whole family.

Learning how to conduct a new patient consultation is one of the great challenges in oncology, and it is particularly demanding in the early years of training when your own knowledge and experience are limited. Very few consultations go entirely to plan and probably the biggest factor weighing against the idealised experience that I have outlined is the pressure on time, especially when you have several new patients to see in the same clinic. You are also a human being, who is allowed to be responsive to pressures on time, on decisions that you have taken about the last patient you saw, on concerns about getting through all the patients you have to see in that clinic, etc. etc. With experience, you will learn how to adapt the time available for the most essential priorities and particularly to judge the level and detail of explanation different patients will require from you. There are patients who will be happy to trust you and will simply answer your questions and accept your judgement; others will want to challenge you on every aspect of your advice. You must learn to strike the right balance in explanation and use of time, satisfying the anxiety and the questions of your patients, but also avoiding giving so much information that the most important messages are lost.

With so much factual information available – on the internet, in brochures, etc. – you can direct patients to reliable sources that complement what you have said at this first consultation (see Chapter 4). Such resources are, however, no substitute for personalised conversation which, above all, should establish confidence in you and in the medical system in which you operate at this early stage of the patient's journey.

The Essential Components of the First Consultation

Plan whatever time is available to encompass the following:

- Study the referral letter and investigations to date *before* meeting the patient.
- Elicit what the patient understands about the reasons for being referred.
- Explain the need for pathology review or staging investigations as necessary.
- Avoid being too specific about prognosis, but do not ignore the issue completely.
- Give the patient an outline of future management.
- Allow time for their questions.

Chapter 3 **Primary Treatment**

In this chapter I offer advice on the sort of language that can be used to explain medical oncology treatment. This treatment involves the use of cytotoxic chemotherapy, hormones, immunological treatments and the newer signal transduction and gene-based therapies.

For some situations – advanced metastatic cancer or "non-surgical" cancer, such as lymphoma – the medical oncologist is clearly the lead specialist, or is the only specialist involved. For many other situations the medical oncologist is part of a multidisciplinary group including surgeons, radiation oncologists, gynaecologists, etc. This applies to many of the common epithelial carcinomas, e.g. breast, colorectal, lung and ovarian cancer, but also to rarer diseases such as sarcomas and malignant melanoma. Multidisciplinary care is now recognised as the gold standard for these situations, but with the added value of combining surgery, radiation and medical treatment and expertise comes the additional complexity of explaining management in an appropriate and coherent way. Your role as the physician in this potentially complex grouping is key to ensuring that patients gain confidence and know who their doctors are. If attention is not paid to this, the patient may feel that they are merely pieces in a complex jigsaw and feel dispossessed. I return to the concept of who is responsible for explaining what and when later, but first let us deal with the basics of explaining medical anti-cancer treatment.

1. Cytotoxic chemotherapy

Cytotoxic chemotherapy has been in routine use for over 50 years. The first successes for such medicine were in the treatment of lymphomas, particularly Hodgkin's disease, and for the treatment of leukaemias – especially in children. The first series of drugs were alkylating agents such as nitrogen mustard and cyclophosphamide. They were soon followed by antimetabolites such as methotrexate and 5-fluorouracil. Despite the enormous advances in our understanding of cancer and the development of many more selective targeted medicines now available, these original drugs are still widely used today. The first generation of drugs were remarkably non-selective in their mechanism of action. I say "remarkably" because they worked – damage to cancer cells exceeded damage to normal healthy dividing cells – hence their continued use. However, this lack of selectivity for the tumour over the host was responsible for the severe side effects associated with their use in the early days of chemotherapy.

Nowadays the knowledge that we have developed regarding optimum dosing and scheduling of these classic drugs, together with advances in preventing important side effects such as emesis and preventing or treating bone marrow compromise, has greatly reduced the toxicity of this type of chemotherapy. Nevertheless, many patients are unaware of such progress and the concept of any form of chemotherapy is still feared by many people. All too often, newly diagnosed patients will assume that any treatment you offer will cause severe sickness, total alopecia and extreme fatigue: this is simply not the case. It is true that the therapeutic ratio (balance between benefit/toxicity) is still narrow for almost all cancer treatments – hence the need for specialised knowledge in their selection and prescription. The essential point is that, in explaining a particular course of treatment for an individual patient, you focus on the side effects specific to those medicines, and dispel (if necessary) false assumptions and fears that in my experience so many patients start with.

Some of the most important advances in cancer treatment over the past 25 years have been in the development of ways to prevent, reverse or minimise the side effects of commonly prescribed anti-cancer drugs. Emesis is the classic example, where the introduction of 5-HT_3 antagonists revolutionised the experience of severe emesis that universally was associated with drugs such as cisplatinum. Classifying drugs into those that cause severe, moderate or minimal emesis allows the prescription of appropriate anti-emetics, and consequently relief from this very distressing problem.

The development of growth factors to prevent, minimise or reverse severe bone marrow toxicity has greatly reduced the incidence of severe neutropenia, with the risk of sometimes life-threatening infection.

Compared with emesis and bone marrow toxicity, we have been somewhat less successful in preventing alopecia. Alopecia is a significant problem for both men and women. Where hair loss is of such magnitude that a wig is recommended, women usually find this more acceptable than men – perhaps not surprisingly, given the rather poorer quality of hair pieces for men. Not all anti-cancer drugs cause alopecia, but some routinely cause total hair loss, and others partial. In most situations hair will regrow – even during continued treatment. When it is appropriate to prescribe drugs that you know will cause alopecia, it is important to counsel patients in advance. Obtaining a wig to match a patient's existing hair colour and style is usually easier if done before their hair has come out. In certain circumstances it is appropriate to use physical methods such as scalp cooling to minimise alopecia. Some drugs (usually analogues of existing medicines) have been developed specifically because they cause less alopecia, just as others have been developed to reduce cardiac or renal toxicities. The choice of which medicine you prescribe for any given patient depends on many factors other than the side effects involved, but where there *are* choices between drugs with similar efficacy, it is important to consider these toxicity issues and discuss the options with your patients.

One aspect of alopecia deserves a special comment. When newly diagnosed or when a relapse occurs, some people will want their families and friends to know – they seek and benefit from their concern at these very difficult times. However, others may not want anyone to know and wish to protect their privacy. Alopecia is one of the few outward signs of something being seriously wrong and, for patients who do not wish others to know of their illness, it will be an added burden if their physical appearance announces this in such an obvious way.

The introduction of inhibitors of epidermal growth factor receptor (EGFR), useful as they are, has produced a new and troublesome side effect – severe skin rash. Usually this affects the face and can sometimes cause severe disfigurement. Similar considerations apply to those mentioned above concerning alopecia. The change in physical appearance with the associated loss of privacy should be balanced with the expected therapeutic gain. You should be sensitive to these issues in reaching an overall decision as to what treatment to recommend.

Neuropathy – sometimes autonomic, but more usually peripheral sensory neuropathy – can develop in patients receiving a variety of anti-cancer drugs. Unfortunately, this is often irreversible and progressive. This problem can be particularly distressing for patients whose work or recreation depends on fine movements of their hands – musicians, artists, seamstresses. Again, the decision as to whether a patient should reduce or stop the causative drug is multifactorial, but an awareness of the risk of developing such irreversible toxicities is important.

This brings me to an important point about monitoring the side effects of all anti-cancer drugs. In situations where toxicities are subclinical – changes in marrow, renal or hepatic function, for example – you monitor by blood tests or other investigations, and the responsibility is yours. For "clinical" toxicities, such as nausea, neuropathy, fatigue and partial alopecia, it is good practice to ask the patient routinely to discuss and report these aspects of treatment. If it becomes part of routine review, it is not seen as alarming or over-inquisitive – on the contrary, it shows concern and is part of holistic care. The earlier you detect significant side effects, the more informed you are about the need for considering an alteration in the management plan.

The timing of when you explain chemotherapy to a patient will vary depending on the nature of the referral and the indication for which you are prescribing. For the management of advanced or metastatic cancer where you are likely to be the only specialist involved, you may have to outline the relevant treatment at your first meeting. This is a particular challenge given all the other information that you are trying to share at the first consultation, and my advice is to be fairly brief if this is the only time to introduce your recommended plan. More often, following the first consultation, staging investigations or further pathology are required and the appropriate time to explain treatment will be at the second or a subsequent consultation – by which time the patient will hopefully be a little less anxious, more familiar with you and the hospital surroundings, and better able to understand, absorb and question the information you are communicating.

Explaining the principles of classic chemotherapy should not pose you any significant problem. Oral medication is clearly understood and most people are familiar with intravenous access, drips and intravenous infusions. If the patient requires a PICC line or central line, they need additional information and, in centres where the chemotherapy is administered by specialised nurses, it may be best to leave the detailed account of the procedure and the relevant care involved to your nursing colleagues. For all patients, the programme becomes much clearer after their first treatment and I have learned from experience that it is both adequate and actually less confusing to keep your initial explanation as brief as possible. It is, however, essential to offer the patient and any accompanying partner the time to ask questions which can dispel myths, reduce anxiety and instil confidence. Above all, when you are still in training, make sure that you are familiar with the acute and chronic side effects of the drugs involved in the regime you are prescribing – it is best to avoid having to consult the formulary or other data source in front of the patient. Remember at all times that you have an anxious patient in front of you and that you are there to reassure and give confidence.

2. Hormone treatment

Hormone treatment – or, more often, anti-hormone treatment – is widely used for diseases such as breast and prostate cancer. These treatments may be given orally or by depot intermittent injection. The side effects are very different from those of cytotoxic drugs but easily explainable and, for most patients, easily understood. The biggest difference between endocrine treatment and chemotherapy is the duration of the treatment, where anti-oestrogens, for example, may be prescribed for women with breast cancer for up to five years, and successful treatment for prostate cancer may involve years rather than months of treatment. The initial explanation of endocrine therapy should include the necessity of this timeframe and, in my opinion, it is never too soon to emphasise the importance of compliance, or adherence as it is now sometimes called. Whereas compliance has long been recognised as a problem with many chronic prescriptions – for hypertension and hypercholesterolaemia – and even short courses of antibiotics, it is now recognised that compliance is an issue for cancer patients, most particularly those on long-term endocrine therapy.

The reasons that patients decide to discontinue treatment of their own volition are multiple. The side effects of anti-oestrogen medicines include hot flushes, dry vagina leading to dyspareunia and loss of libido. Men with prostate cancer taking endocrine therapy have to be helped to accept the impotence and loss of libido associated with this, but do not underestimate the significance of the chronic fatigue that can greatly reduce the quality of their lives whilst on treatment. Good cancer care is all about good communication between you and your patient; if you have succeeded in establishing a trusting relationship with your patient, then you should encourage them to discuss the quality of their lives on treatment, and any wish that they might have to adjust or discontinue treatment, so that they understand the benefit/risk of any decision that you take together. Starting out on endocrine treatment is straightforward; living for long periods of time on treatment presents a real challenge for some patients. With the passage of time, you will be assessing the degree of benefit obtained and discussing the side effects of treatment, and this will inform your own subsequent advice about the need to continue or possibly modify treatment in one way or another. The essential factor is to explain to patients right at the beginning of a protracted course of treatment the need to take their medication as prescribed or, if they struggle with this, to come and discuss the situation with you in a positive, non-threatening, friendly and supportive way.

3. Immunological therapy

For a long time scientists have been researching the relationship between cancer and a patient's immune system. This relationship is highly complex. Whilst it is not thought that failure or dysfunction of the immune system causes cancer, it is now believed that altered immunity can facilitate or promote the development of cancer once the process has begun. Patients often ask if their immune system has failed or is "not working properly", and I usually answer this by explaining that the immune system is part of our "housekeeping" machinery. In full working order, it is one of the body's processes by which damage (in this case, malignant cell division) is recognised as being "wrong" and for certain cancer processes the immune system is activated, the rogue cells destroyed and the process arrested before a clinical cancer develops. Where the immune system is impaired, this policing does not take place and the cancer develops.

If cancer can be promoted by a faulty immune system, it was a logical step to try to develop anti-cancer therapies that restore efficiencies in the immune system or boost it in some way. Early trials with totally non-specific immune stimulants such as bacille Calmette–Guérin (BCG) were unsuccessful, but in recent times greater understanding of the complexity of immune surveillance and the interplay between the tumour and its host have led to some successes.

The cytokines, alpha interferon and the interleukins, are used to mount an immune response against certain forms of cancer – for example, renal cell cancer and malignant melanoma. If you are prescribing courses of these agents, you will have to explain something of the above-mentioned interaction between host and tumour, and the principle of administering these substances by intramuscular, subcutaneous or intravenous injection over a period of several months or even years. The major side effects of both of these cytokines, and indeed many forms of immunotherapy, are short-term fever, but more significantly long-term fatigue – sometimes to a very severe degree. This is especially the case if high doses are prescribed, as is still fashionable in the USA – although much less frequently used in Europe. Patients need to be warned about this to prevent them making the assumption that these symptoms are caused by their cancer progressing and that this is what is sapping their strength.

Very recently we have seen the development of much more specific immunotherapies than those of the cytokines referred to above. The identification and characterisation of tumour-specific antigens has enabled the development of molecules such as ipilimumab, which has proven active against malignant melanoma, and cell-based vaccines such as sipuleucel, which is active in prostate cancer. Both of these products are associated with specific side effects which must be explained to patients. The success, at long last, of developing specific immunotherapies has given a real boost to this area of cancer research, and it is likely that other specific anti-tumour immunological treatments will be developed in the near future.

The term "anti-cancer vaccines" is one that I prefer to use only very selectively. One of the most important developments in the field of immunological therapy in recent years has been the development of "true" vaccines against the herpes virus family responsible for carcinoma of the cervix. By "true" vaccine I mean the prophylactic use of this vaccine before a young woman has been exposed to the antigen, and hence to stimulate the development of immunity in the same way as for the classic viral infections of childhood. I do not like the use of the term "vaccine" for immunotherapies to treat established cancers – where clearly the antigen has failed to produce a natural antibody response or at least in sufficient amounts to prevent the onset of cancer. However, this term is frequently used for describing all immunotherapies and you should be prepared to answer any questions that patients may pose to you if they are confused by the term "vaccine".

4. Gene-based therapies

Research to investigate the human genome has identified an awesome array of genes and molecular pathways that are involved with the growth, proliferation and survival of cancer cells. Unfortunately, with few notable exceptions, very few such genes or pathways are unique to the cancer cell. It follows that, despite this knowledge leading to an unprecedented number of new potential treatment molecules being developed, the holy grail of true selectivity, i.e. killing only the cancer cell without harming the normal counterpart, still eludes us. Even more frustrating is the realisation that having developed therapeutic molecules which prevent a given gene from producing its protein, or blocking a particular pathway involved in driving the cancer, the tumour can divert to an alternative set of genes, or bypass the blocked pathway using another route to sustain its growth. This process leads to what we recognise clinically as drug resistance, usually associated with disease progression.

The science behind these recent developments is referred to as "signal transduction". By this is meant the series of processes by which a metabolic signal, received by a specific receptor on the cancer cell surface, sets off a chain of chemical reactions transmitting or transducing that initiating signal to the nucleus of the cell. Consequently changes in gene function within the nucleus will either prevent the production of a given protein on which the cell is dependent for its survival, or may promote excess production of a growth-promoting protein leading to cancer growth.

The pharmaceutical industry has invested enormous sums of money in developing signal transduction inhibitors and these are now widely available. Many of these new treatments are small molecules that enter the cell to interfere with its chemical machinery and are prescribed as oral pills or as an intravenous injection. Resulting from the same scientific research, monoclonal antibodies have been developed that block the receptor on the cell surface, thus preventing the initiating signal. Monoclonal antibodies are usually administered intravenously.

The mode of administration of signal transduction inhibitors and monoclonal antibodies is similar to that of the older cytotoxic drugs, but their side effect profile is somewhat different. Many of these compounds – for example, EGFR inhibitors (as mentioned above) – cause skin rashes that can be very distressing to patients, but ironically this usually reflects that the treatment is working. Other signal transduction inhibitors cause very debilitating diarrhoea and some cause selective organ dysfunction, as in the cardiotoxicity associated with Her2 inhibition used in the treatment of breast cancer.

You have to explain the relative balance of benefit to risk with these less familiar medicines and of course, as with all conversations explaining treatment to your patients, it is essential that you are familiar with the specific side effects of the medicines that you are prescribing – and confine any given conversation specifically to these.

5. Explaining the purpose of treatment

Whilst it is obvious to you what you hope to achieve in prescribing a particular treatment plan for a patient, it is important to appreciate that the specific goal of treatment may not be immediately obvious to your patient. It is not uncommon for a patient to ask early in a first consultation, "Is my cancer curable?" For many people, cancer is regarded as either curable or untreatable. They may or may not know the answer to this question and may be testing you as to your openness, but how you answer is critical to the whole ensuing management. In the rare instances of cancers such as testicular cancer and some lymphomas and other low-volume epithelial cancers, you may be able to offer a reasonable chance of cure. However, for the vast majority of patients, the objective of medical treatment is to reduce symptoms, control the cancer during a period of remission and prolong life. How you approach the explanation of this depends on the reasons for using medical treatment. For the patients presenting with advanced metastatic epithelial cancer – colorectal, lung, breast, etc. – the objectives of treatment are to reduce the size of the tumour, thereby reducing symptoms, and to slow or stop the progression of the disease, thereby enhancing general health, appetite, energy, mood, etc. to improve or maximise the quality of a patient's life for as long as possible.

In my experience it is never too soon to introduce patients to the concept of the different phases of their illness, as referred to in Chapter 1 – a period of active treatment followed hopefully by remission, but often later by recurrence. Many patients find the concept of remission without cure a very challenging one – living with a "time bomb" inside them, and this is discussed in Chapter 5. This anxiety is partially relieved if patients are taking medication continuously during remission, such as happens with endocrine therapy in breast and prostate cancer, but this is also relevant to the concept of adjuvant treatment.

"Adjuvant treatment" is the use of chemotherapy and/or hormone therapy after primary treatment with surgery or radiation. Courses of treatment are typically given for four to six months, with the aim of destroying any of the malignant cells not eradicated by the primary mode of treatment but that are undetectable, as illustrated in Figure 1 in Chapter 1.

Patients starting on adjuvant treatment following surgery – for example, in breast or colon cancer – will still be recovering from the consequences of that surgery and now have to cope with the additional burden of the side effects of chemotherapy. When you explain the need for this "systemic" treatment, it is important to be positive about the potential for long-term benefit, without creating added anxiety about the fact that cancer cells may well have escaped from the primary site, even though they do not show up as tumours on scans, etc. I do not like the expression "belt and braces" as used by many physicians, and you should avoid using phrases that suggest a guarantee of cure or long-term survival by the use of adjuvant treatment. The challenge for you and the patient is that in the adjuvant setting there is no clinically obvious disease to follow and your prescription relies on statistical probabilities rather than the individual's response to treatment. Most patients find it helpful to have this explained to them.

The term "neo-adjuvant" has been coined to describe the situation when patients receive chemotherapy (or occasionally endocrine treatment) as a prelude to surgery. Again using breast cancer as an example, the administration of two to four courses of chemotherapy prior to surgery may significantly reduce the scale of operation needed – a mastectomy may be avoided in favour of a lumpectomy, or the cosmetic result of a lumpectomy may be facilitated by reducing the size of an initially very large tumour. The great advantage of neo-adjuvant treatment is that the pathologist can give an accurate report of the degree of response for an individual patient when the resected specimen is analysed. This allows you to individualise any subsequent post-operative adjuvant treatment in a way that is much better informed than in the case with conventional adjuvant treatment. When the pathologist confirms a good response to treatment, you have a very reassuring message to convey.

Explaining adjuvant and neo-adjuvant systemic therapies should not pose any specific difficulties for you as the medical oncologist, but it is important to establish which members of the team of specialists say what and when to the patient. As already mentioned, we now accept that in many situations patients receive the optimum treatment if they are managed by a multidisciplinary team. This is, however, potentially confusing for patients and it is important that you establish with your colleagues who will explain each part of the process, work-up, treatment and subsequent assessment, and particularly when this information is to be given. If you take the example of ovarian cancer, the patient will usually start in the care of a gynaecologist, who will establish the diagnosis and resect as much tumour as possible at the initial operation. The patient is then referred to you for chemotherapy and may or may not require further surgery later. The condition is treatable but, with very rare exceptions, incurable. Having had the privilege of working with excellent gynaecological oncologists who genuinely enjoyed sharing the care of their patients, I established the process whereby the gynaecologist would be the first person to confirm the diagnosis to a new patient, but would not discuss prognosis or any detail of the medical plan until we had reviewed the case together in a multidisciplinary conference, and agreed a management plan that I would then explain to the patient and their family. In this way there is a seamless handover from surgeon to physician and the patient can be helped to have confidence in all the people involved in her care. I have had other much less fortunate experiences where new patients are referred by surgeons who have apparently told the patient that they are being referred to medical oncology either for "belt and braces" to complement the surgery or, worse still, "to be cured"!

The message here is to establish with your local colleagues an appropriate division of labour regarding the explanation of what is to happen next, and importantly which specialist will explain this and when. Done well, the patient gains in confidence – done badly, confusion can be really harmful. These multidisciplinary aspects are discussed further in the next chapter.

Chapter 4 Communication within the Context of Multidisciplinary Care

Modern cancer care requires the integration of many different professional groups, oncologists (medical, radiation and surgical), haematologists, gynaecologists, urologists, etc. etc. Nurses play a pivotal role and, where they are available, psychosocial oncologists can be of great value to all concerned. The patient is the central focus of all this communication, but, with access to the web and patient support groups, many patients find themselves confused by too much information, and sometimes have too little time to absorb and digest it before having to make key decisions about their management.

In this chapter I offer some advice about the importance of awareness. As the oncologist, you have the primary role in designing and explaining management plans, but it is very important that you are fully aware of the input from colleagues in other medical disciplines and from your nursing colleagues, and of the information and advice that patients have gathered for themselves – from the web, patient support groups, etc. In Chapter 3 I referred to the issue of communication with medical colleagues, but in this chapter I want to illustrate specific inputs from nurses, psychosocial oncologists and patient advocacy/support groups.

Oncology nurses

It is impossible to overstate the importance of good communication with your nursing colleagues. The development of oncology as a specialisation within nursing has revolutionised the experience of so many patients, and it is important that during your training in oncology you learn to understand and appreciate the role that oncology nurses play. In my experience, patients relate to nurses in a different way than to their doctors. However friendly, open and compassionate the doctor appears, many patients need to keep a respectful distance from the doctor, who they see as having the primary role in the decision processes regarding their management. On the other hand, nurses are often perceived to be more accessible for sharing concerns and uncertainties about what is happening to a patient at any given time – this is most particularly seen in the outpatient setting. Whilst patients are in hospital, good doctors will make the time to talk and listen to their patients, but it is inevitable that, in the clinic, time is always a pressure. Of course this also applies to nurses, but where there is good communication between you and your nursing colleagues, the additional input from nurses can add inestimable value for both you and the patient.

I have been most fortunate in having excellent clinical nurse specialists (CNSs) attached to each of the disease-specific clinics in which I have worked. To follow the CNSs' own assessment of new patients, and to share the information gathered about specific aspects of their disease, symptoms, anxieties, aspirations, and family and work pressures, can greatly enhance your decisions about management. Patients often confide such anxieties much more freely to a nurse than to a doctor. In my experience, patients will often ask the nurse rather than the doctor what to actually expect during treatment, and this gives the nurse the opportunity to re-explain and amplify information that you may have given during your consultation. In my practice the CNS would give each new patient a card with their contact details, and encourage patients to use this whenever they wanted to resolve specific queries at the time that they were troubled. Few patients abused this availability, but many patients have reported to me that having this contact information in their purse or wallet was hugely reassuring.

Another area where good communication between doctor and nurse can benefit everyone concerned relates to clinical trials. Apart from the obvious need to conduct clinical research, it is well established that patients benefit from enrolment in trials. Nevertheless, as I discuss in Chapter 7, many patients are initially nervous, and the amount of detail in consent forms can be overwhelming. Nurses can play a vital role in encouraging enrolment to trials by helping patients to understand what is involved, and reassuring them of the extra attention that inevitably results from trial participation. Similarly, nurses will often help to retain patients on trials, when doubts about the value of continuing cause anxieties that the patient may not wish to expose to their doctor. Nurses can also play an important role in monitoring adherence to medicines. In the days when nearly all oncology treatments were administered intravenously, adherence was not an issue. However, with the increasing use of pills, often to be taken for very long periods of time, we are becoming aware that some patients may either become forgetful or make a definite decision to stop taking their medicines. It is a patient's right to do as they please, but it is essential that the doctor knows what is happening. In my experience, patients are more likely to tell the truth to a nurse than risk the wrath of the doctor, if they admit to having ceased taking their medication!

These are but a few examples of the need for you as the oncologist to work closely with your nurses, so that, with their help and input, you are as fully informed as possible of the patient's attitude to their illness at the different phases thereof.

Psychosocial oncologists

The development of the speciality of psychosocial oncology (PSO) has brought a new dimension to the holistic care of patients with cancer. As a discipline, PSO has developed with input from psychiatry, psychology and nursing. Unfortunately not every oncologist has access to psychosocial oncologists, but it is to be hoped that this will change in the years to come. For those of us who are fortunate to have such colleagues, it is essential that good communication is in place to optimise this very valuable resource. Where it is available as part of the team in which you work, then there is no excuse for poor communication, but you may have to refer outside of your institution or, in some circumstances, patients may be able to self-refer. In these situations you must make every effort to ensure good communication between both sets of professionals and the patient. As with my comments on the nurse's role above, since this is not a textbook or manual on the totality of cancer management, I will focus on three aspects where I believe good communication between you, the oncologist, and colleagues in psychosocial oncology is particularly relevant.

Patients

Not all patients need to be referred to clinical psychologists, and where you have access to a psychosocial oncologist it is important in your training years that you learn which categories of patient are most likely to benefit, or who to discuss with your PSO colleagues when you are considering a referral. A common theme throughout this entire book is your role in helping to reduce anxiety and give confidence to patients who have such a life-changing diagnosis as cancer, with all that that implies. There is considerable demand for psychological medicine in the day-to-day practice of oncology, but you must learn to detect and refer those patients for whom specific PSO support is required.

Such patients are those who appear to have exceptional levels of anxiety or depression that are not being adequately managed by yourself or the patient's family physician. Clinically significant levels of anxiety and depression are not an inevitable sequela of cancer, but as oncologists we must learn to recognise patients suitable for referral to specialists in the talking therapies, for which there is now a strong evidence base. By gaining their own specialist understanding of cancer, the psychosocial oncologist can help patients to understand the reasons for their severe anxiety and depression, and address contributing issues such as the guilt that can be associated with carcinogenic lifestyle factors – for example, cigarette smoking, excess alcohol consumption, sexual practices, obesity, etc. Exploring such issues may then help patients with their relationships with partners, children, family, friends, work colleagues, and so on. For those patients who need such support, the development of coping styles will usually be of great benefit in helping them to tolerate anti-cancer treatment and the episodes of recurrent anxiety that occur during follow-up in remission. Good communication between the psychosocial oncologist and you will therefore give you very useful information about the optimal way to manage the oncological component of your patient's care.

Medical and nursing teams

Psychosocial oncologists can make a major contribution in helping the medical and nursing teams to look after cancer patients. I refer briefly in the Epilogue to the demands made on oncologists over a lifetime of working with cancer patients. This is very challenging medicine, and there are times when all of us feel emotionally drained by the narrow margin between success and failure in cancer care. In my own centre, we found enormous help from our psychologists in supporting the medical and nursing staff – either collectively or individually. Communicating over a specific patient's problem often exposes issues for doctor or nurse – either about that specific patient or more generally. The opportunity to discuss this and seek help from our psychosocial oncologists in understanding patients and our own attitudes to them or their circumstances has often had a profound effect in helping staff with their own coping styles. As individuals, seeking the help of a psychosocial oncologist at a time of difficulty should never be seen as a personal weakness, but rather as evidence of professional maturity. Working as a team, there are times when there is a collective sense of undue stress leading to low morale – maybe a run of very challenging patients, a particularly sad death, or the loss of a key member of staff for any reason. At these times, input from a psychosocial oncologist who knows the team as a whole can be very beneficial.

Research

There is an ever-increasing interest in research into psychosocial oncology and it is important for oncologists to be aware of the way that they can contribute to this. A classic example is the difficult area of Quality of Life (QoL) studies. A variety of instruments have been developed to assess QoL, but the uptake of them is still very variable. Where these studies relate to the assessment of new drugs, for example, they can, when used well, make a significant contribution to the controversial area of assigning a value to "effectiveness". Used badly, they only create noise in the system. Whilst oncologists usually agree on criteria that describe the side effects or risks of novel treatments, there is much more controversy about the "benefit". The traditional measures of overall survival or progression-free survival are less useful than they used to be, now that so many drugs are being developed for chronic administration over several years. In these situations, the quality of a patient's survival may be at least as important as life expectancy – or even more so. Psychosocial oncologists have a pivotal role in designing the measures required to assess this, and we as oncologists must be aware of our role in referring patients for such studies, and understanding what is involved.

Patient support groups and the internet

The creation of patient support groups (PSGs) offers invaluable support in many ways. The ability to share anxieties and uncertainties, to learn from the experience of others, and to have people to whom to turn for advice and comfort who are not immediate family or dependents are very powerful aids – especially to newly diagnosed patients. Some PSGs operate on a national or even international basis, providing literature and information for individuals, and lobbying on their behalf for funding, research, greater awareness, etc. Other PSGs operate on a local level to provide direct support to patients. PSGs are usually aware of the positive aspects of participating in clinical trials, and may be helpful to both patients and researchers in encouraging enrolment into trials. As an oncologist, it is important to be aware of which PSGs are appropriate and available to your patients and, most importantly, to discuss with patients their use of such facilities. This is in no way intrusive on your part, but reflects your concern to encompass every aspect of holistic care.

Most aspects of interaction between your patients and PSGs will be positive, but there are a few potential pitfalls of which you should be aware. As an oncologist, you recognise the subtle but important differences between subsets of patients with apparently the same diagnosis. Increasingly we are stratifying these subsets because they have different prognoses and therefore need different approaches to management. I have had numerous experiences of patients being confused and often upset by advice offered from fellow patients which was intended to be helpful, but did not in fact refer to their specific problem.

Obtaining misinformation is a real risk with the increasing use of the internet by patients seeking to obtain as much information as they can, especially early on but also at critical times, such as at relapse. Some websites are excellent and very helpful – especially those run by or informed by knowledgeable PSGs. Unfortunately there are other sites that are out of date, promotional in one way or another, or too superficial to be of real value.

In this book I often refer to the obvious challenge of time. The patient needs as much as possible – in consultation with you and the other professionals and whilst researching on their own before having to make key decisions. Unfortunately time is always against us for the key face-to-face encounters. In recent years I have been increasingly frustrated by the need to use precious time during consultations in unpicking information that the patient has obtained for themselves, which is inappropriate to their specific circumstance. The patient enters your consulting room brandishing pages they have downloaded from a website that they have confidence in. There is a positive message about new research, new drugs or diagnostic processes, or a revised prognosis, perhaps. You have to peruse this literature as rapidly as possible and you realise that it is either irrelevant to the specific situation of the patient in front of you, or wrong, or refers to a research study suggesting benefit, but the intervention – typically a new "breakthrough" drug – is not yet available. It takes skill and experience to handle the ensuing conversation so that you do not instantly depress your patient, completely destroy their self-confidence, or dismiss their completely understandable desire to obtain as much understanding as possible of their condition. The worst aspect of such encounters is that you are using up invaluable time for communicating the information that *is* relevant to this particular patient.

The use of self-acquired knowledge is likely to increase in the future and, hopefully, so will the quality and accuracy of the information available. The positive aspects of this are to be welcomed and, as oncologists, we should do whatever we can to assist in developing good web-based sources of information and to help reduce the negative ones. In the same way, we should interact with PSGs to optimise the overall exposure of patients to an ever-increasing if sometimes confusing knowledge base. It is all about good communication.

Chapter 5 **Explaining Follow-up**

The term "remission" means different things to different people. As the doctor, you understand the concept of successful treatment to reduce the size and metabolic behaviour of the tumour such that the disease is no longer clinically detectable and the symptoms have resolved. As referred to in Figure 1 in Chapter 1, we are, however, aware of the biological fact that all too often some residual cells remain in the patient, dormant for weeks, months or years, but which eventually regrow to emerge as a clinical relapse. For the patient, remission means successful completion of therapy, a much hoped for freedom from illness and, even amongst the most intelligent and well-informed patients, a glimmer of hope that perhaps the disease will never come back. As the medical oncologist, you have a responsibility to explain your assessment of the relative success of primary treatment and the purpose of monitoring patients over the months and years ahead. Let us consider firstly the assessment of tumour status at the end of treatment and then your approach to follow-up.

In the past, I used to believe that patients would be universally pleased to get to the end of the four to six courses of treatment typically prescribed for an epithelial cancer. Whatever the degree of side effects and after the complete or partial disappearance of symptoms and signs of cancer, I assumed that all patients would be glad that treatment was completed – at least for now – and that they would only have to return to the clinic for occasional follow-ups. Careful research has shown that, for many patients, the period immediately following the time of completing their treatment is associated with new anxieties and loss of confidence. The drama of diagnosis and the "busyness" of treatment with its frequent attendances at the hospital is suddenly replaced by a void – no-one asking questions, less external care and, for some, a newfound aloneness with their condition. Life has changed because they developed cancer, but where are they to go now, how should they return to a "new" normality, practically and emotionally? Only the patients themselves can decide how to live their lives under the new situation of being a cancer patient under follow-up, but having been treated. Whether or not to return to work, how much exercise to take, whether they wish to change other lifestyle activities such as diet, etc.? Only they can make these decisions, but you can be of enormous help to patients at this vulnerable time by anticipating some of this uncertainty in the period of transition from active treatment to passive follow-up.

When seeing patients to discuss your assessment of the degree of benefit they have gained from primary treatment, it may be helpful to explain that it is not at all uncommon to feel a sense of abandonment and loneliness, now that they are not required to come back to the hospital so frequently. I have often advised patients to be kind to themselves, particularly at this time, and not to rush into full rehabilitation too quickly. Taking exercise is good for all of us – but punishing yourself in the gym every day may be too much, too soon for many patients. Dietary fads may reveal themselves and patients may often seek your approval for ways in which they can take some control of their health in a manner that they were unaccustomed to before their illness. I discuss possible advice about complementary medicines in Chapter 8, but be prepared for questions about alcohol, food, exercise, sexual activity, family relationships and work-related issues. Your patient will be greatly helped if you find the time to support and encourage them at this particular time. The degree of interest that you show in the totality of their lives will inevitably help them through the next phase of follow-up surveillance.

Monitoring remission

Medical progress has created some new problems for both patient and doctor in deciding the optimum way to follow a patient's health once the primary treatment period is over. Beyond the help referred to above in the immediate post-treatment period, you have to decide how often to review your patient and what tests or monitoring devices to use. It is for the multidisciplinary team of professionals to decide how and when it is technically sensible to monitor subclinical disease or to look for markers that anticipate relapse. Different diseases warrant different approaches. For example, for some cancers it makes little scientific sense to look for tumour regrowth if there is little by way of subsequent treatment to offer, whilst for other tumour types the detection of relapse at the earliest moment may impact the benefit of second- or third-line therapy.

Whatever the monitoring programme for an individual patient, it is essential to explain to them the rationale for recommending a particular blood test, X-ray or scan. Never assume that the patient will just "expect" such surveillance, and remember that every time you do a monitoring test you will create anxiety for the patient – to be beneficially relieved if all is well, but dismayed if the results are negative – as discussed in the next chapter. So my recommendation is "never assume" and "always explain". Outline your local policy for monitoring disease during remission and ask if the patient is comforted by the positive aspects of reassurance or otherwise. I have had patients for whom the severe anxiety of monitoring their disease has truly ruined the quality of their lives during remission. The constant reminder that they had had cancer, and were still at risk of recurrence, was so stressful for them that we stopped monitoring them altogether and awaited clinically obvious signs or symptoms of relapse. Other patients need the reassurance of constant monitoring of their disease status. Good communication and caring enquiry into your patient's mental and emotional state, as well as their physical symptoms, at follow-up visits will allow you to help your patients to gain the best that they can out of the time spent in remission.

Two specific situations require comment. The first is self-monitoring and the second is the use of biomarkers. I have often been asked by patients what they should look out for by way of symptoms or signs that might herald a relapse. My usual answer to this has been to suggest that if I were to detail the complete list of symptoms that *could* be relevant, they will start to experience some or all of them on the way home from this hospital visit! With rare exceptions, I discourage patients from a daily self-enquiry of everything that might be abnormal and try to help them trust the system of monitoring in place at the hospital, unless of course they develop specific signs, such as haemoptysis, haematuria, melaena or such like. My emphasis is to try to demedicalise their lives as much as possible, whilst they are clinically in remission.

The continued search for biomarkers is adding new complexities to the monitoring of subclinical disease. As we find more and more subtle ways of detecting tumour reactivity – proteins released into the blood or urine, metabolic imaging technology, circulating tumour cells and so on – the greater is the scientific ability to know whether a patient's tumour is relapsing. But is the use of these new technologies beneficial to the patient? The use of CA125 monitoring in ovarian cancer is illustrative. Unfortunately the measurement of CA125 in the blood is expressed in numbers – numbers that patients ask for, write down and remember. Many ovarian cancer patients will attend a follow-up visit and the first question they ask is, "What is my CA125 today?" Research has shown that detecting relapse of ovarian cancer by means of CA125 measurement gives a three- to four-month lead before the woman becomes symptomatic. This, however, is of little value in terms of benefit from second-line treatment. Conversely, the emotional impact of knowing that clinical relapse is about to happen can be devastating, and the period of "disease-free" survival is curtailed. Research is unstoppable and it is difficult to argue that, as clinical scientists, we should not wish to know as much as possible about what is happening to our patients. Nevertheless, the continued development of more and more sophisticated ways of monitoring patients is likely to lead to more time being required from you, as the oncologist, to interpret results in an individualistic way, taking into account all of the holistic features of living in remission referred to above.

Relapse

Explaining to a patient that their disease has relapsed is one of the hardest medical challenges that you will ever face. If accepting a diagnosis of cancer is devastating to most patients, being told that their disease has come back may represent the very worst moment in their entire experience of the disease (see Figure 2 in Chapter 1). The reasons for this are not hard to understand. Throughout my professional life I have admired the way the vast majority of patients accept a diagnosis of cancer. Awful as this moment is, very few people "go to pieces" and, whether facing this alone or supported by family, most people find their own way to cope with the processes of staging, work-up and treatment. If you have done your job well initially, the patient will have developed trust in you and your professional team and found a coping strategy that allows them to get on with their lives, albeit in very different circumstances. Whatever they felt emotionally during the initial shock of diagnosis, and whatever information was conveyed and received by them, many patients settle to an optimistic attitude that they will overcome their disease and that it will remain at bay.

All of these positive elements are destroyed when relapse occurs – potentially a loss of confidence in you and the whole medical profession, but above all a loss of self-confidence: everything that they were trying to do, every adjustment that they had made to their lifestyle has all been a waste; everything is useless, the future is unbearably bleak. Your role is to try to restore these confidences – and, where appropriate, to explain that there are other treatments to consider. Without being patronising or creating false hope, you should try to reassure your patient that life is not yet over, and that you and your team are fully committed to the next stage of their care. Above all, do not try to cheer the patient up, or dismiss their distress by suggesting that this is just a natural progression of their illness. You will almost certainly have known all along that relapse was likely or a certainty, but you will not have known when this was going to happen. Understanding that this is emotionally the lowest point for them will help you to empathise with patients and help them come to an understanding of the next phase of their illness.

How a patient learns of their relapse is of course key to all of the above. In many instances the patient does not need to be told – they have already worked this out for themselves. For some, there are obvious signs: losing blood from the gastrointestinal tract, in urine or through coughing will inevitably alarm a patient. Seeing new pigmented lesions on their skin may be an obvious event for a patient with melanoma; swelling of lymph nodes may be obvious to a patient with lymphoma, etc. Other more subtle changes – anorexia, significant weight loss or abdominal swelling – may cause sufficient concern that the patient seeks an early review.

In these situations, my advice is to be immediately straightforward, and as open and honest as possible, recognising the huge impact on the patient of confirming their worst fears. Where it is immediately obvious to you that relapse has occurred, you must say so and begin the conversation to discuss the consequences. The manner in which you speak will be influenced by your patient's likely prognosis. Where there are realistic possibilities of further useful treatment, you can sincerely introduce positive elements – not to dismiss the seriousness of the relapse, but to explain further options that may avoid a sense of hopelessness which can make it very difficult for patients to make *any* decision about more treatment. In situations where you feel that there are no further active measures to be pursued, you have to introduce the concept that attention now needs to focus on palliative care – symptom control and psychological/emotional support. The process is harder if you need to carry out investigations to confirm a suspicion of relapse and that, of course, introduces a delay and additional anxiety for the patient, until you can explain what is to happen next.

The situation is a great deal more challenging if there have been no prodromal symptoms or signs to warn the patient, and it is you who finds or suspects relapse at a routine review. If you have to explain this "out of the blue", it will require all of your communication skills. How often patients have studied my face as I examined them or their scans or blood results – looking for concern, doubt or anxiety in my facial expression. Many people have written advice on how to break bad news and I accept that there are some guiding principles – I am offering some on these pages – but in the end you have to develop your own way of doing this. It does get easier with experience, but it is always difficult and draining of your own emotional resources. The setting for such sensitive conversations is critical. A quiet outpatient consulting room is ideal, providing privacy and at least a little time for the patient to absorb what you are telling them. For an inpatient in hospital, there is the potential advantage of having the opportunity and time to explain over more than one conversation, but privacy can be hard to achieve in many hospital ward settings. In either circumstance, I advise you to take your time – by which I mean that you do not have to explain everything at once: how you diagnosed relapse, what options there are for further treatment, what is the likely prognosis, etc. The explanation that their disease has recurred may be all that the patient can cope with initially, and all other information may go unheard or, worse, may confuse and add to distress for both the patient and their family. It is sometimes best just to confirm the relapse and leave it for a subsequent conversation to discuss further options. The most important thing is to be clear – do not evade the issue, especially when confirmatory investigations are needed. Try to empathise with the inevitable distress experienced, whilst at the same time offering a clear message of support, be that active (further treatment) or passive (palliative care). Never is there a time when patients have a greater need of your confident support, but at least initially, while you are training and developing your skills, never will there be a time when you feel more exposed.

One of the most difficult situations that we have all faced during training is when you suspect relapse but realise that this is going to come as a complete surprise to the patient in front of you. You may not yet have the knowledge base to know the full range of further management options or to answer the patient's and their family's questions. Honesty is the key to their confidence, and it is entirely appropriate for you to explain that, whilst you suspect or have to confirm that their disease has relapsed, you will have to seek advice from your senior colleagues as to the most appropriate course of action to follow. In assisting trainees in this situation, I have often received compliments from patients and their families as to the way in which the young doctor conducted him or herself in explaining relapse and its consequences.

Patients will respect your honesty and openness in seeking advice and, far from diminishing, their confidence in you will increase. Asking advice from colleagues is of course not something confined to training. I have often explained to patients that I wish to discuss their situation with colleagues, or take time to consider things on my own before formulating a management plan to propose to them. When patients realise that you are considering every aspect of their care on an individual basis, they are reassured and appreciate that they are not just progressing from one protocol to another in a formulaic way.

Explaining further management options

For the newly diagnosed patient, when you are explaining your initial treatment plan, you will often have to discuss different options. Long gone are the days when the doctor simply told the patient what was going to happen next. For primary treatment, you will usually have a strong preference for which treatment you recommend and your goal is to explain this within the context of possible alternatives, but guiding your patient to the treatment that you think best suits the situation. The circumstances of choosing the optimal management plan for relapsed disease are more complex.

Where initial treatment is based on an institutional protocol or your "standard" approach, you are making a recommendation on the basis of statistics and probabilities. When patients ask about their prognosis at this time, I often explain that for them, as an individual, statistics are of little help and that it will be more appropriate to discuss prognosis after we assess their response to treatment; by that time, their case is individualised and prognosis much more accurate. When considering options for second-line treatment, you have the knowledge of whether primary treatment achieved a good result, a moderate result or was of little value. Clearly your approach to future management is going to be greatly influenced by this knowledge. Before explaining your options to the relapsed patient, you need to consider the following:

1. Is there a case for re-treatment with the same initial programme?
2. Are there second-line treatments likely to be of benefit to your patient?
3. Depending on 1 and 2 above, you have to decide what you are hoping to achieve for your patient now that they know their disease is incurable.
4. Is there a role for research or experimental treatment?
5. Should you forego active treatment and focus only on symptom control and quality rather than quantity of life?

In some situations (usually following a lengthy period of remission), it is appropriate to re-treat the patient with the same therapy that they have previously received. This situation is not difficult to explain, and your major challenge is to help patients to cope both with their disappointment that the disease has recurred, and with the knowledge that they will have to go back to regular hospital visits, needles, infusions and any side effects that they experienced before.

If there are second- or third-line treatments that are regularly used in the situation your patient now finds themself in, it is important that you identify a clear purpose in prescribing such further treatment. Patients should not receive any treatment just because it is available, and, most particularly when making decisions at relapse, you will frequently be dealing with patients – and their families – who have lost confidence in the purpose of any further active treatment. If you know from experience that there is a reasonable chance that your patient will benefit from second- or third-line active treatment – in terms of relief of symptoms, improvement in general wellbeing or life expectancy – then you will choose a management plan accordingly. You must then discuss not just the specifics of drugs and schedules, but above all the reasons why you recommend this further treatment.

One of the challenges that you may face quite frequently in recommending further treatment is when there is a difference of opinion between your patient and their spouse, partner or closest family members. It is not at all uncommon for the patient to be reluctant to embark on further treatment and yet the family are desperate for them so to do. The patient is demoralised, depressed, feeling hopeless and helpless and cannot see the point of having to tolerate further toxicities for possibly little or no benefit. The husband, wife or children, however, are desperate to leave no stone unturned and to persuade their loved one to try any and all means of staying alive for as long as possible. This situation requires skill and tact. You are the only person in the room who knows the scientific probability of benefit versus harm, but also the one who is not emotionally responsible for the consequences of whatever decision is reached.

My advice in this situation is as follows; your first responsibility is to your patient. You have to assess to what degree he or she has benefited or suffered from treatments so far, and assess as best you can how much more therapy they will tolerate. Naturally this is balanced by the nature of the cancer and the likelihood of a second or third significant remission – in which case, accepting that some short-term toxicities may be acceptable. Similarly, even without inducing a further (partial) remission, you may feel that active anti-cancer treatment is the best approach to resolve the symptoms and signs of their illness. Your second concern is the patient's family. If patients have previously been accompanied by their closest family members when attending clinics, you will have had a chance to gauge the dynamics of their relationship to a greater or lesser extent. Care, affection, concern and anxiety for their loved ones is the natural reaction displayed by most people, but spouses of patients can be very angry too. Spouses can be genuinely angry that they are going to be left to cope with life on their own as a result of the patient's cancer. Loneliness and anxiety about coping with everyday life, housekeeping and financial worries all come into the picture. You are the patient's doctor, not the family's counsellor, but it is important to develop the skills to assess family dynamics and tensions, most particularly when you are trying to help everyone involved to choose the best way forward. Try to make time to listen to the family's wishes, try to help them understand your reasons for recommending active or passive treatment at this stage, and try to help those involved to avoid argument and divisiveness when they are no longer in your presence. How you explain the options and the goals of any specific second- or third-line treatment plan will have an important impact on both the patient and their family later in the course of the disease. In some situations the patient may ask you to speak to their family separately, to explain the situation under circumstances that spare the patient further tensions within the family.

We live in an age when doctors are increasingly expected to explain options, but you should avoid at all costs being too directive in recommending any specific choice. I fully support the concept that, providing the choices have been explained in an appropriate manner, it is for the patient to decide which plan to follow. However, there are situations where I believe it is a part of our professional responsibility to help patients by leading conversation that directs them towards a particular path. In this situation, where a patient and their family are confronted by the dual challenge of disappointment that the disease has progressed and the need to make a decision on what to do next, it may be very difficult for them to reach *any* decision. If you have a strong feeling for what is most appropriate from the medical/scientific point of view, then it is often very helpful for you to say so. It is possible to be authoritative without being overbearing.

Seeking a second opinion

Many of the messages in this book are offered to help you gain confidence in your communication with patients – to help you create and sustain an air of trust that enables patients to have confidence in you and the team of professionals around you. Even when you achieve all that you could wish for in this regard, given the extreme importance of making the right decision about treatment – by you, your patient and their family – it is not surprising that some patients may seek a second opinion, either initially or particularly at the time of relapse. Indeed, there is an increasing trend to encourage this, especially from patient advocacy groups (see Chapter 4).

Patients seek second opinions for a variety of reasons. For example, you may have offered a choice of options involving different possible outcomes – balanced by different levels of toxicities, or inconveniences. The latter might be, for example, an inpatient regime versus an outpatient treatment. Or you may have explained that in your opinion no further active treatment is appropriate. By understanding and reflecting on the reasons for seeking a second opinion, you will learn to accommodate and, where appropriate, facilitate such, without becoming defensive or taking this as any form of personal criticism. Think how often we all seek second or multiple opinions before choosing a phone, computer, car or a holiday destination. It is part of everyday intelligent life. Perhaps it is surprising that not everyone seeks such plurality of advice when confronted with choices for cancer treatment, but that probably reflects a need to have confidence and trust in *someone*. If you have done well in that regard so far, patients may not want to take the additional time involved in seeking a further opinion. Similarly they may be anxious not to appear to be ungrateful to you. The latter point has nothing to do with flattery – it reflects their need to feel that you will continue to do everything appropriate for them to the best of your ability, not risking the idea that you might consider them to be an "awkward" patient.

So my advice is simple. When confronted with a request to seek a second opinion, I advise you to react positively and in a manner that demonstrates your understanding of their need for confirmation or otherwise. If the second opinion results in a totally different management plan, the patient may transfer to someone else's care, and you must accept this graciously. If the result, as is more usually the case, is to confirm your plan or to select an option from a choice that you gave, then the patient's confidence in you is enhanced and is in no way undermined.

Clinical trials

It is not unusual for patients relapsing for the first or a subsequent time to be eligible for clinical trials or experimental therapy. By definition, research involves the unknown, and introducing elements of uncertainty requires great care – most especially at the time of relapse, when patients may find any decision-making difficult, and even more so if there are conflicting ambitions between patient and family. How you explain research to patients is discussed more fully in Chapter 7.

If your recommendation is that there are no reasonable further active anti-cancer treatments to pursue, or if your patient and their family decide not to pursue further active treatments, then the focus of management is symptom control and issues affecting the quality rather than the quantity of the patient's life. In some medical settings this will remain the responsibility of the oncologist, but in others this may involve specialists in palliative care and this is discussed in the next chapter.

Chapter 6 **Progression and Terminal Care**

In the previous chapter I suggested some ways that may help you in explaining to a patient that their disease has relapsed, and issues to do with subsequent active treatment where that is appropriate. Let us now consider your role in helping people come to terms with the situation where further active anti-cancer treatment is inappropriate – where progression is going to lead to terminal care and death. When you have gained the confidence to talk openly with patients about these issues, you will find it rather less difficult than some earlier conversations that you have held, and profoundly rewarding. The major reason why these conversations are more straightforward is that there is now much less doubt, less confusion, less choice for the doctor and fewer decisions for the patient to make. As a constant theme throughout this book, I have emphasised that one of the greatest challenges that patients with cancer have to face is the uncertainty of what lies ahead. At this stage of the disease many of those uncertainties have passed. It is now your role to focus on the relief of physical symptoms and to offer appropriate emotional and psychological support to the patient and their family. Your aim is to help all of those involved to reach a peaceful state as they prepare for the patient's death. Let us first consider your role in treating physical symptoms at the time of progression.

Managing physical symptoms of advanced cancer

Considering the whole of cancer management, one of the greatest achievements of recent years is the progress that has been made in managing the physical symptoms of advanced cancer. We now understand the causes of pain, nausea, vomiting and fatigue, for example, and this understanding has led to new treatments and plans of management. Whilst of course not confined to the management of symptoms, this new knowledge has made a major contribution to the recognition of the medical speciality of "palliative care". Within the medical profession there can, however, be confusion about the language we use to encompass medical oncology, palliative care and supportive care.

To play your part in the optimum care of a patient with advanced cancer beyond the phase of active anti-cancer intervention, it is essential that you establish which colleagues in your environment are responsible for which elements of management. No one misunderstands the oncologist's role in the active phases of treatment, but the interface between oncology and palliative care can lead to confusion, and even cause distress for patients and their families if this is not clearly explained to all concerned. The name "palliative care" comes from the Latin *palliare*, meaning to cloak – implying a hiding of the distress of symptoms such as pain, without influencing the underlying cause. Some people mistake the role of palliative care, relegating it to the short period preceding death, but specialists in this discipline have much to offer at earlier stages of a patient's illness, in the same way that oncologists should not be regarded as "chemotherapists", only concerned with the earlier active anti-cancer treatments. I use the term "supportive care" not to refer to a medical specialism but to the practice of using medicines to alleviate symptoms such as pain, fever and emesis at any stage of the illness. Medical oncologists are trained in the use of such medicines and their correct use plays a vital role in obtaining the optimal value from anti-cancer drugs at any stage of a patient's illness.

Where oncologists have to practice without the professional support of palliative care specialists, they must extend their supportive care repertoire to the pre-terminal and terminal phases of the illness. More fortunate oncologists who have the benefit of working with colleagues in palliative care need to establish at what stage and how to transfer care from the one to the other. This concept of a seamless transfer of care is absolutely key to the support needed by your patient and their family. You must avoid at all costs the perception that your role as the oncologist is now over, and "all that is left" is palliative care. At the appropriate time, when you have decided that no more active treatment is appropriate (or of course if the patient has chosen that path), and the patient is developing symptoms that could benefit from the input of specialists in palliative care, you should explain the reasons for introducing your colleagues and effect a transfer of responsibility in a way that reassures your patient and their family, rather than implies any sense of abandonment and hopelessness. The patient should feel that you are calling in all the resources available to you to optimise their continuing care. In the situation where palliative care specialists "visit" a patient in your ward or clinic, it is important that you establish who is responsible for what, and most essentially that the patient knows this. In the situation where the patient transfers all their medical care to palliative care, for example by moving to a hospice, or only returning to outpatient attendances at a pain clinic, etc., it may be difficult for you to continue to contribute to that patient's care. However, when it is possible for you to visit a patient in a palliative care ward or hospice or even at home, as I have sometimes been able so to do, this can have a huge impact on the patient and their family by experiencing your continued interest in their care.

Management of pain

Of all the symptoms that cause difficulty for both patients and the medical profession, it is worth making some specific comments about the management of pain. For a variety of reasons this particularly important symptom is often managed poorly and yet the knowledge and skills are available to improve this situation greatly. Many patients inappropriately assume that a diagnosis of cancer will automatically lead to pain and eventually a painful death. Even at their first consultation, patients have not infrequently asked me if they will have to suffer from (uncontrollable) pain. There is no question that many malignant diseases do cause pain, especially as they advance – bone metastases would be an obvious example – but our knowledge of the causes of pain and therefore how to manage this very important symptom has revolutionised outcomes.

As an oncologist, you must acquire not only the skills to manage pain but the ability to explain this to your patient. When you achieve this successfully, you will enhance the value of the medication, not least by reducing anxiety, a pain enhancer, but also ensuring compliance with your prescription.

Sadly, many patients and their families have a reluctance to take strong analgesics, particularly opiates, for fear of addiction – an entirely inappropriate anxiety in advanced and terminal illness. Even more distressingly, this attitude is still held by some doctors and nurses. Modern pain management depends on three cardinal features, as illustrated below.

Essentials of Pain Management

- Accurately assess the cause of pain.
- Prescribe correct analgesic for the specific type of pain.
- Use sufficient strength and quantity of pain medication.

The causes of pain as experienced by any individual may be complex and so each of the above three factors should be explained to the patient, for reassurance both that you understand the problem and that you have a management plan to address this. Most importantly of all, ensure that the patient adheres to that plan. The four-step analgesic ladder (Figure 3) illustrates the need to escalate analgesia as required from mild to strong treatment, depending on the severity of the pain experienced.

The latter changes with time, and you will need to re-evaluate patients frequently if pain is a severe problem. At these reviews you can reassess the causative nature of the problem, especially the positive or negative effect of emotional factors that may be contributing to the problem and that often change with time (see below). Above all, you must persuade your patient that taking sufficient pain relief, and taking it regularly, is not only allowed but essential to your ability to help them. In the management of severe pain, the aim is to use sufficient, regularly administered analgesia to keep patients pain-free or as pain-free as possible.

Figure 3: Four-step analgesic ladder for stratified use of analgesic therapies.

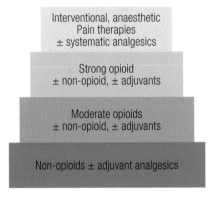

Interventional, anaesthetic
Pain therapies
± systematic analgesics

Strong opioid
± non-opioid, ± adjuvants

Moderate opioids
± non-opioid, ± adjuvants

Non-opioids ± adjuvant analgesics

Emotional and psychological support

At no time in their entire illness will patients benefit more from your medical skills than when you are able to offer emotional and psychological support at the stage when their disease is clearly progressing towards the terminal phase. In helping patients transfer from the "active" phase of treatment to an acceptance that they are now nearing the end of their journey, I often refer to the idea of chapters in a book. The stage of progression represents a new chapter in their book, not necessarily the last one but nearer the end than the beginning. You should explain that the time has come to recognise a different objective from the management plans that you have explained earlier in the course of their illness. You wish to focus with them on improving physical symptoms and, more than ever, to offer emotional and psychological support. The very fact that you want to engage your patient in conversation, especially listening to and discussing their anxiety and fears, is itself of enormous comfort to most patients. One of their greatest fears at this time is that you will abandon them – that you have done as much as you can during the active phase of management and that all that is left now is death, and a potentially lonely one as well. Learning how to offer empathy in a non-patronising way for patients at this stage of the illness is really important. You cannot learn this from books – you can benefit from observing more senior and experienced colleagues, but essentially you have to find your own way to do this. Environment, tempo, language and physical elements such as touch are all relevant here.

Environment

When the purpose of a consultation is to inform your patient that their illness has reached the stage where you no longer recommend active anti-cancer treatment, or if it is time to prepare them for the last chapter in their personal book, the environment in which you hold such a conversation can have an enormous bearing on the patient's response. Privacy, quietness and comfort are the key elements. Such conversations (and I include those with family members here, either with or without the patient present) should never take place in public corridors or busy hospital wards. Of course, I accept that sometimes a hospital ward is the only place available, but even then, if at all possible, try to have the patient moved to a quiet space, ideally a separate room. Quietness can be an elusive goal in a hospital setting, but I am describing the ideal situation for which you should aim. By "comfort" I mean that you should endeavour to have the patient seated or supported in the most comfortable position achievable, so that they can concentrate on what you are explaining, and respond in as dignified a way as possible. If patients feel particularly anxious at this time – anticipating that you are about to deliver bad news – then anything that helps them to preserve their dignity is important, and the environment in which such conversations are held contributes an important part to this.

Tempo

By tempo I mean not only the speed at which you talk, but the timing of the whole conversation. It is important to allow sufficient time within these conversations for the message to sink in, and for the patient to have time to formulate an appropriate response. If a patient is fully expecting what you are about to say, it is likely that their first reaction will be to question you – asking how certain you are of the situation, exploring alternatives or asking direct questions about life expectancy.

If this message is a surprise, it is not unusual for patients to lose their self-control temporarily and to cry – this may also be the response of accompanying family members. In this situation, you must allow time for them to recover their composure before you continue or they begin to question you. The speed at which you talk is important since, if you go too fast, it is not only harder for the patient to absorb fully what you are saying, but it implies that you are in a hurry and have more important things to attend to. In reality, you may indeed be very pressed for time, but the speed with which you converse and your body language must attempt to create a sense of peacefulness and calm that will greatly help the patient and their family.

Language

In all conversations with seriously ill patients, it is important to choose language which is clear, non-confusing, avoids technical phraseology or jargon and is appropriate to the person with whom you are conversing. It is surprising how often doctors, especially those in training, forget this. The easiest messages to understand are ones that are given in a clear, simple and honest way. This does not imply a short blunt statement, left unqualified. You may know the patient in front of you quite well, or not at all, but you can judge from their demeanour how much they may be expecting the message that you are about to deliver. If your tempo is right, you allow them time to absorb the message in stages – not necessarily all in a single statement. In the process of wanting to provide some comfort, it is very common, especially for less experienced doctors, to follow a statement of bad news with immediate "qualifiers" to try to soften the blow. By "qualifier" I mean statements such as, "Of course, we do not know when this is going to happen" or "Sometimes the unexpected can occur". My advice is to be very careful in using any qualifying statements that detract from your main message, at least until you are certain that your patient has understood the essential facts and future plans of management.

At all times you are seeking to reassure your patient that you are there to help in a professional way, in whatever capacity; they are not alone with their problem and you are every bit as concerned with their health now as you were at the beginning of their illness. In days gone by, there were stories of doctors who seemed to regard irreversible or untreatable disease as some sort of personal failure or slur on their professional competence – hard to believe nowadays, but sadly true. The fact that your patient's cancer is progressing does not represent any failure on your part, and your patient will not blame you for the situation in which they now find themselves. On the contrary, if you show empathy, understanding and compassion, you are making an essential professional contribution at this critical time. Anyone can learn to diagnose cancer and select appropriate treatment policies – that is the science of medicine. It is much harder to learn the art of empathy without being patronising, of showing compassion for the sadness of the situation and giving reassurance that the patient will be cared for right up until the inevitable end.

It may be helpful to comment on the use of the word "truth" and the telling thereof. It can sometimes be challenging if a patient or their closest family members confront you with the phrase, "Please, doctor, tell me the truth". Your initial reaction to this might be to be somewhat affronted, as if they are implying that you have not been fully open and honest all the way along. Do not take umbrage at this, but recognise that, to give honest and open answers to questions, we must distinguish between the concept of a "true statement" and "telling the truth". By this I mean that you must distinguish between factual accuracy and veracity, i.e. telling the facts, such as they exist, honestly and without altering (softening) their meaning or withholding vital parts of the story. Just as I have suggested great care with offering qualifying statements to soften the impact of bad news, so it is just as important to avoid euphemisms or other non-direct ways of explaining your message. This is most particularly important when you have to discuss imminent death, as discussed later.

Physical touch

Whilst this book is essentially about conversations and ways to explain cancer and its management, it is important to remember that your own physical demeanour plays its part in the way in which patients can be helped by your explanations. Just as I have suggested that environment and tempo are important for delicate conversations, so your own behaviour is of course important. However busy a day you are having, however much you have to deal with multiple, simultaneous demands, it is essential for the conduct of these most important conversations that you find the inner resource to appear calm and composed and to behave as though time is of no consequence. Conveying the concept that you have all the time in the world can provide extraordinary comfort to patients in this situation; so too can appropriate physical touch.

Patients in the advanced stages of cancer feel isolated and alone, not only emotionally and psychologically but also physically. As illness advances, partners, family members and friends physically withdraw to the extent of not even touching them at all. Shaking hands becomes a light touch on the elbow, a proper kiss becomes a peck on the cheek, and everyone seems to forget the value of a real hug. (Woe betide the doctor who speaks to his patient from the foot of the bed!) Touch is a form of communication, and in the process of conducting the most sensitive conversations it is of great value to establish physical contact between you and your patient. In the consulting room, I always greet patients with a handshake – often using both hands. Resting your hand on the patient's forearm whilst conversing helps to convey an added sense of concern. Similarly, when talking to patients at the bedside, holding their hand or resting your hand lightly on their forearm can add a seemingly disproportionate value to the sense of care and concern that is experienced by the patient. As part of good care for patients towards the end of their lives, there is great value to be gained from the use of physiotherapy and gentle massage that involves sensitive touch – fulfilling one of life's basic human needs. Let us now turn to the ultimate conversation – talking about death.

Talking about death

In helping people prepare for death, you are no longer "explaining" cancer, but sharing your professional skills in talking about what ultimately awaits us all. Where there may be little left to explain about cancer, your professional knowledge and experience of having helped others prepare for death can provide an invaluable comfort to your patients and especially their families. As your own skills and comfort zone mature, with experience you will find that helping people to confront their own impending death becomes easier. In the early years of practising oncology, it can be a real challenge to know what to say and how to say it. Whilst death is uniquely personal, we are more similar than we are different. There are areas of common ground that you should seek to understand when developing your own way of talking with and listening to dying patients. The one cardinal rule is not to avoid the issue: do not shy away from talking about death – at any time when a patient raises the issue, but most especially when the patient understands that the end is in sight. It is absolutely not our role as professionals to try to "cheer people up", to create a false sense of hope or, even worse, to dismiss people's anxieties about death by avoiding the issue.

There are some basic rules that you should appreciate to help you develop your personal approach to this. In her landmark publication entitled *On Death and Dying*, published in 1969, Dr Elisabeth Kübler-Ross described five stages of a process by which people cope with the impact of being told they have a terminal illness. These five stages are:

1. Denial

2. Anger

3. Bargaining

4. Depression

5. Acceptance

A great deal has been written about Kübler-Ross' model, some supportive and some critical, but in my own experience there is real value in reflecting on the message that she conveyed as a framework on which to develop your own approach.

The concept of initial denial is indeed common – both at diagnosis of cancer and at the stage of being told that active treatment is no longer appropriate. Denial is especially prevalent in the situation where the patient has no new symptoms. Progression of their disease may be identified medically by a radiological scan or a set of blood tests, for example, and, feeling no different, the patient simply does not want to accept the bad news that you have delivered. Denial does not usually persist for any length of time and your role in this phase is to hold fast to the truth that you have explained, and be sympathetic as you wait for the patient to realise that what you have said is sadly true.

Anger is hardly surprising – especially when your patient is young or far from the age of normal life expectancy. "Why me?", "Life just isn't fair", "What have I ever done to deserve this?" – an entirely understandable response to unacceptable news. Your role is to recognise this anger, which may be railed at you as the purveyor of bad news, or against the spouse, partner or family. By recognising this emotional response and explaining that it is entirely natural, you offer support to both the patient and their family through a passage that can be profoundly distressing. This is especially the case when close family and friends are trying to offer help and support, but in return only experience rejection.

Bargaining is more subtle than denial and anger. By bargaining, Kübler-Ross refers to the way in which we all seek to promise something in return for avoiding the unacceptable – in this case, death. So we try to reason that if we agree to some changes in attitude, lifestyle or religious belief, then we will deserve a prolongation of life, a postponement of death. Rekindling of religious beliefs is not unusual in this situation. Depending on your own religious beliefs, or lack of them, you may or may not feel able to support a given patient through the turmoil often associated with this aspect of bargaining. Heavy smokers who are dying from lung cancer know that it is too late to stop smoking, but the concept of this sacrifice may represent for them a bargaining token for life extension. Attempts to resolve previous family tensions may be used in bargaining – either from the patient or a family member. Your role is to be aware of the concept of bargaining, thereby not missing opportunities to offer sympathy, support and sometimes practical advice (since you are not directly involved in the family conflict). Simply allowing patients time to ventilate their bargaining strategies may provide comfort, and diminish the sense of loneliness that sets in as the bargaining strategy fails.

Depression is hardly surprising, but it is not an invariable accompaniment to the preparation for death. Depression is not the same as sadness, which for the vast majority of people is an entirely natural feeling at this stage, most especially for those who have led a full and rewarding life, or of course for those dying at an inappropriately young age.

In my experience, when patients are nearing death, they are often aware of this themselves. Being the most natural thing in life after birth, it is hardly surprising that as the body ceases to function – for whatever reason – our minds perceive what is happening physically. We have made good progress in our ability to relieve the distressing physical symptoms of terminal illness – pain, dyspnoea, restlessness, constipation and nausea, for example – but as death approaches many patients will recognise a sense of fatigue bordering on exhaustion and realise that the end is not far away. If your patient achieves a state of physical and emotional calm and is aware of what is happening, then you have done your job well, and there is nothing left to explain except to maintain honesty about what is happening. Relatives will nearly always ask if death is imminent, but on many occasions I have been asked directly by patients, "Am I dying?" If it is clear to you that this is indeed the case, then my usual reply would be to say, "Yes, I believe that you are". The response then is usually to say, "Thank you for being so honest". Again, this openness transmits professionalism and reinforces to the patient that they are not alone and that you are still involved and caring for them.

The situation is straightforward when you know that your patient has only a few days or a week or two to live, but is more difficult at a previous stage, perhaps one to two months earlier, when death is inevitable but the exact timing is uncertain. At this stage I always try to avoid being too specific. Phrases such as "probably only a few months" are honest in describing a short outlook, but are perceived differently from the true final phase, of which, as I have said, the patient is usually self-aware. You must be prepared for potentially awkward questions – designed not to test your medical knowledge but to test your openness and honesty. "Do you think I should book that holiday next summer?" "I must be able to get to my granddaughter's wedding in six months' time". The patient is studying your face and observing your body language to test whether you think that they have one month or six left. If you are prepared for such challenges, my advice is to repeat whatever has been said previously about prognosis (denial may still be happening) and explain that both you and the patient "will have to see how their health changes week by week in the months ahead". These conversations have to be individualised and there is no set programme to follow, but the best help that you can offer your patient, and especially their family, is to be as straightforward as possible, not condescending or patronising, but to engage all those concerned in the conversation by reflecting your genuine continued interest in their situation, and to share their sadness in a professional way. Above all, do not dismiss the topic because it makes you feel uncomfortable.

Students and those who have had little or no experience of helping dying patients often ask about fear – are dying patients afraid? In my experience, sometimes people *are* genuinely afraid, but for the most part the great majority are not. Nevertheless, if you suspect a sense of fear, it is important and very relevant to ask if your patient is afraid, and therefore "of what?" Is it fear of the unknown, fear of the process of death, fear for the safety and wellbeing of loved ones who will be left? You should be prepared to ask about these and listen to the answers. Many of these fears can be allayed, but only if you create the opportunity for them to be aired and discussed.

Bereavement

Much has been studied and written about the emotional and physical consequences of losing a loved one. As a practising oncologist, you may or may not work in a setting where there are structured bereavement services. Sadly, many institutions do not provide this, but as an oncologist you are only one of several professionals who may be involved in helping relatives come to terms with the death of a close family member or friend. As the doctor involved in providing active anti-cancer treatment and helping patients and family to prepare for death, it is not uncommon that the last direct contact you have with relatives is at the moment of the patient's death. You may have had the chance to get to know the closest family members quite well during your patient's final illness, and in my own experience, in cases where I have not had the opportunity to be involved in their subsequent bereavement, it has left an unsatisfactory sense of incompleteness in your holistic management of the patient's overall illness. Time is always in short supply in professional life, and caring for the living will take precedence over care for the families of deceased patients, but sometimes there are unresolved issues about your patient's illness that still require explanation and discussion. Questions such as, "Why did such and such happen?", "Did we (that is you, the patient or the family) make the right decisions about X or Y (to change treatment, to stop treatment, to try something new, etc.)?".

In the days before we had the investigative capacity that now exists, we frequently had to rely on post mortem autopsies to reach a final medical conclusion about the illness. In that situation, a meeting with family members was often necessary to deliver the relevant explanations. Nowadays there are fewer uncertainties prior to death and autopsies are requested less frequently. However, if time permits, there will be occasions when offering to meet bereaved relatives will not only help them significantly with their new situation and with moving forward in their own lives, but can also bring a sense of professional completion to your role as an oncologist. Two aspects of this are particularly important to understand – timing and place.

Timing

It is recognised that there are certain moments in time which are especially important in the grieving process. The first comes approximately six weeks after a death. At this time the bereft person is beginning to recover from some of the acute grief reactions – weeping, tearfulness, exhaustion, sleeplessness, anorexia, acute anxiety about day-to-day activities – and is beginning to learn how to cope. However, at about six weeks they can be struck with a sudden sense of loneliness and abandonment. Our explanation for this is that many people find, at about this time, that their closest family, friends, neighbours, colleagues at work, people they meet in the street, etc. have all expressed their sorrow, have offered some emotional or practical support, but feel that they cannot continue to enquire after the bereaved's wellbeing and, quite understandably, need to get on with their own lives – not as though nothing had happened, but just because it is the nature of society that "life continues". For the bereaved, this apparent loss of daily caring enquiry can emphasise the sense of loneliness and loss that overwhelms them, and can make it even harder for them to pick themselves up and start to re-engage with the world around them. If you are counselling a bereaved relative at about this six-week time point, it can be helpful to explain the vulnerability experienced by many people at this time, thereby reassuring them that their behaviour is normal, understandable and in no way reflects a lack of care from the people with whom they come into contact in their daily lives. As with many states of emotional distress, time is important in the healing process, and you can reassure the bereaved that, with time, they will progress through this period of depression and extreme sadness to a period when they can more happily reflect on the positive times with a loved one, whose loss they now experience so strongly.

The second time point of which you should be aware occurs approximately six months after death. Our understanding of this is less certain, but it is commonly found that at about this time many people will experience an acute depression and recall the feelings that they previously experienced at the time of their relative's death. You are much less likely to be directly involved in counselling the bereaved six months from the patient's death, but being aware of this vulnerable time point may help you to offer advice at the earlier stage, gently warning that at about six months' time there may be a recall phenomenon that again will pass in due course.

One of the reasons for explaining this is that, where it is appropriate, you may wish to warn the bereaved against making any life-changing decisions too soon: for example, selling their house, changing jobs, taking retirement, etc. etc. – lest important events should coincide with this six-month dip in the recovery from a loved one's death.

Place

If you do decide to meet with grieving relatives a few weeks after a death, the physical setting for that interview is important. In the past I have made mistakes by inviting relatives to return to the clinic room where I previously used to review the patient. The process of trying to help the bereaved move on can be set back by the physical reminder of a consulting room associated with the patient's illness. Where possible, it is better to meet relatives in a new space, an office or meeting room which provides a more neutral surrounding, which from experience I have found is more comfortable for the grieving relatives. As with so much of the process of helping patients and family to understand and cope with cancer, attention to the small details of where such meetings are held can have an extraordinary effect on the benefit obtained from such conversations.

Much of the advice offered in these pages concerns ways in which you, as the expert, can reassure an anxious patient and their family that medical knowledge and expertise can help them both physically and emotionally to cope with cancer. From your expert knowledge and previous experience, you guide your patient through the investigations and advice on treatment that you consider most appropriate at different stages of their illness. I have emphasised that an open, honest, caring approach will comfort an anxious patient and reassure them that the future is not a frightening, blind abyss. Prognosis is not a certain science, but hopefully you have created a sense of trust and reassurance that you and your medical team know what you are doing.

Research is an integral part of cancer medicine. The progress made in recent years is evidence of the value of this, but our outcomes are still very far from acceptable, especially for many of the common cancers. Nowadays research embraces every aspect of cancer from fundamental cell biology to genetics, epidemiology and the study of risk factors, markers of tumour behaviour and, of course, clinical trials. Some of the most useful research has concerned supportive care – both physical and emotional. A lot of this is in the public domain and many patients will be aware of the value of research and certainly of the need for research. So why do I include a chapter on explaining research to them? The answer is that research – especially clinical trials – involves "uncertainty", the very thing that you have been trying to avoid, resolve or help the patient to accept. So explaining research is really important.

There are many different settings in which you may find yourself having to explain a research study. We increasingly recognise the vast complexity of human cancer; for example, we now appreciate that there are many subtypes of common cancers – breast, lung and colorectal cancer are no longer considered single diseases and, whilst the concept of truly personalised medicine is far off, we are increasingly able to categorise patients into subgroups for whom specific treatments are most appropriate. These new classifications have resulted from the study of biomarkers, which may be assessable from blood but more often require tumour tissue. Explaining the concept of harvesting such tissue by biopsies that are additional to standard procedures should not present you with any particular difficulty. Similarly, if a research study requires additional staging procedures, scans or biopsies, it is usually straightforward to explain the science behind the question, and the specific procedures involved. The real challenge comes in explaining the concept of clinical trials. A straightforward phase II non-randomised investigation of a new medicine, new dose or new schedule should not be difficult to explain. However, the randomised trial can present real challenges where you have to help patients retain their confidence in you, but you need to explain the unknown outcome of a test between a conventional versus novel intervention or, even more problematic, novel intervention versus placebo or best supportive care.

There are some basic principles concerning the explanation of research that can help you to order any conversation when suggesting that a patient may wish to participate in a research study. We may think of these as benefits versus risks.

Benefits to the patient

Particularly concerning participation in clinical trials, there is a significant body of evidence to prove that patients benefit from taking part in research. The major factor here is that enrolment in a protocol-driven trial assures the patient that every detail of their pathology, staging and eligibility and, of course, treatment is going to be carefully checked and monitored. This gives added assurance to the "quality control" of their care. Participation in a trial often involves additional tests to monitor progress – which may be reassuring – and the additional care involved from medical and nursing staff can bring extra comfort to patients. Depending on the nature of the trial, there is also the added anticipation that their outcome will be improved if new medicines or schedules prove to be superior to conventional treatment. The most obvious benefit is when such anticipation is fulfilled by positive improvement.

Risks to the patient

The very fact that you are explaining a research study introduces the dreaded "uncertainty" again. When explaining a clinical trial, you must remember to explain that research questions do not arise "out of the blue", and are not in any way whimsical ideas, but are based on rigorous science, pre-clinical testing for efficacy and toxicities, and, depending on the nature of the trial, a varying amount of prior experience in other patients. Patients are never "guinea pigs" being experimented on out of curiosity; they are partners in a carefully designed and controlled research environment, where a relevant question is being addressed in as thorough a way as possible. Nevertheless, you have to explain that the outcome is uncertain, otherwise you would not be asking the research question.

Participation in clinical trials may involve additional visits to clinics or even inpatient stays, and some patients may not want the hassle of this – especially if life expectancy is short. Studies of tumour markers may require additional biopsies or blood tests, response assessments, extra scans, etc., all of which may be perceived as negative intrusions.

Sometimes exposure to new medicines causes unexpected side effects, and even expected or familiar toxicities will often be experienced in a research setting, whilst the patient derives little or no benefit from the treatment. Clinical trials which randomise patients between a new treatment and placebo have their own difficulties. Scientifically such trials are often particularly useful in giving a clear-cut answer to the benefit versus risk of a new intervention, but understandably most consenting patients hope that they will be randomised to the active treatment group. Where such trials are blinded or particularly double-blinded, the explanation is much easier, but where this is not the case you must take extra care in explaining the value of the question being addressed, and giving the reassurance that if you *knew* that the new intervention was an improvement you would be prescribing it, not conducting the research. Similar problems exist in explaining trials that randomise a new intervention against best supportive care. Again, my advice is to emphasise the value of the trial (addressing an unanswered question) and the necessity for a control group, giving the assurance that patients so randomised will indeed receive your "best" supportive care.

The concept of hope – true and false hope – straddles both benefit and risk considerations in explaining research to patients. It is understandable that however carefully you have explained the trial treatment and addressed the uncertainty of outcome, many patients will build up a sense of hope that receiving something new is not only going to work but will add real value to their health. This sense of hope can be truly beneficial, especially in the setting of relapsed disease or when conventional treatments have been exhausted. However, the degree of hopefulness may be unrealistic (false hope) and, whether at progression or when standard treatments have run their course, there is a reflex downside if and when the new treatment is seen not to bring benefit to an individual. As the oncologist, you must be prepared for this and willing to talk to disappointed patients, re-explaining the reasons for conducting the trial and reminding them that the outcome of research is by definition unknown – this is challenging medicine.

Helping patients to feel hopeful when explaining a research study is not only allowed, but is good medicine – one time when you can turn uncertainty to advantage, i.e. the patient may benefit from the unknown. However, the degree to which you encourage a positive attitude must be tempered by the potential consequences of the disappointment (hopelessness) that may follow if the new intervention is not successful.

The concept of Informed Consent is extremely important, but is not always addressed in the intended way. Many research studies are accompanied by written explanations to help patients not only to understand more fully the nature of the particular research study, but to help them formulate questions that will better inform their choice as to whether or not to participate. Such written material is very valuable, but is not a substitute for a clear explanation from you, tempered to the previous experience of your patient, their level of medical/scientific knowledge and the influence, helpful or otherwise, of their family.

Where the patient has been informed by you of the existence of a relevant research study and, by inference, has your recommendation that participation would be appropriate, it is essential that they are given adequate time to assess the information, read any relevant material, and then be given the opportunity to pose questions concerning issues that may be unclear. Where clinical trials are concerned, it can be very useful if practical details of treatment are explained by a research nurse after you have initially outlined the basis of the study, as discussed in Chapter 4. Not only are nurses expert at conveying practical details of investigations and treatment, but patients often feel more relaxed in conversation with a nurse, in ways that they may not feel when talking to you as the doctor. However good your communication skills are, patients may be shy to ask specific questions about practical details and may be particularly concerned not to disappoint you, as their doctor, if they wish to decline participation in the study, but fear that you will then have less interest in their subsequent care. Obviously that is not the case, but it is a commonly held concern.

One final comment on the issue of hope versus the reality of uncertainty. In order to defend against disappointment or even criticism in an increasingly litigious environment, some doctors lay too much emphasis on the possible negative outcomes of research, i.e. they over-emphasise the unpredictability of an individual's likelihood of response to a new intervention. The balance between this over-cautious attitude and one of creating a sense of hopefulness by trying something new is a matter of judgement; it depends on the patient and it depends on you. If you know the patient well, you will have some anticipation of their likely willingness and enthusiasm or otherwise to participate. You must avoid "promoting" a research study in a way that will embarrass the patient if they wish to decline, but at the same time avoid the over-cautious emphasis on the potential negatives.

Phase I – First into Man studies

A very particular form of explanation is necessary for the discussion of phase I or First into Man studies (FIMS) with cancer patients. In the early days of medical oncology, almost everyone became engaged in phase I studies, but nowadays these are usually conducted by sub-specialists practising in major research centres. Whether or not conducting such studies yourself, all of us may be involved in referring patients for such research, and therefore it is necessary to have an understanding of what is involved, especially to appreciate the subtle benefits for patients in these "non-therapeutic" trials.

Currently there is much debate about the best way to plan and conduct FIMS with new anti-cancer agents. The classical phase I trial sequentially enrolled very small cohorts of patients (typically 3–6), who were exposed to increasing doses of drug until toxicity occurred. This was essentially a human toxicity test – usually accompanied by clinical pharmacology studies to ascertain knowledge about maximum blood concentrations, duration of action and mechanisms of metabolism and excretion. Different schemes for dose escalation have been used, but typically the initial doses would be very low (for safety reasons) and therefore very unlikely to yield any useful therapeutic response for the individual patient. Towards the end of such phase I studies, when administered doses would be producing measurable signs of toxicity, one would look for "hints of activity" in order to plan the subsequent phase II trials, where looking for efficacy is the key objective.

Many of the recently developed agents with potential anti-cancer activity do not result in toxicities predictable from linear dose escalation. Often there is a given exposure of these drugs (dose and schedule) which is optimal in terms of anti-tumour effect, but where further dose escalation adds only toxicity without additional anti-tumour benefit. For these agents, the use of imaging techniques – of tumour and sometimes of the drug itself – and biomarkers of anti-tumour effect offer the possibility of designing FIMS in a more sophisticated way than the above-mentioned classical dose-escalation concept. It is to be hoped that this new approach will result in fewer patients needing to be exposed to sub-therapeutic doses of a trial medicine, and equally importantly in more rapidly identifying optimal doses and schedules of new drugs to progress to full anti-tumour assessment. Whichever type of phase I/FIMS you are involved with, there are two essential elements to consider – firstly, the choice of patient and, secondly, the way that you explain the purpose of such trials and their risk/benefit ratio, which is different from any other clinical trial.

Not all patients are suitable for inclusion in FIMS and it is therefore essential that you embark on conversations/explanations about such trials only with the appropriate individuals. The usual starting point is that, for any given patient, either they have exhausted the known active treatments or there are no known useful options – an increasingly infrequent situation now that we have active drugs for tumours such as malignant melanoma and renal cancer, which were considered highly refractory to any anti-cancer medicines until fairly recently. In considering patients who have progressed through known treatments, it is important both for the patient and for you to consider life expectancy. To gain useful information from a FIMS, the patient must live long enough for an adequate assessment of the drug–tumour and drug–host interaction. Even though the primary aim of such trials is not the potential anti-cancer effect, it is obviously a useless experiment if the patient does not survive long enough for adequate assessment of organ toxicities – bone marrow, gastrointestinal tract, skin, etc. etc. – and usually this requires more than one exposure to the new drug.

Special consideration applies to the exposure of patients to new drugs if they have known organ compromise – impaired hepatic or renal function, for example, or severely compromised bone marrow function from previous therapies. Inclusion of such patients may be very informative for assessment of the pharmacokinetics and pharmacodynamics of the new drug, but extra care must be taken when enrolling such patients, in order to ensure that their lives will not be foreshortened from the side effects of the drug being investigated.

These considerations about life expectancy are not simply a scientific matter to secure the completeness of the trial. Obviously putting any patient at inappropriate risk is unacceptable, but it is also a matter of ethics – it is unethical to enrol any patient into a trial if their involvement cannot contribute knowledge to the question being addressed. Judging life expectancy is never easy, but the essential point here is to try to avoid discussing phase I/FIMS with patients for whom you judge life expectancy to be too short for either them or you to benefit from their participation.

So how do you explain a FIMS to an appropriate patient? The basics are simple: new medicines come from laboratory science via toxicology – usually involving animals – to the stage where their effects have to be tried in man. For many medicines these FIMS are conducted in healthy volunteers, but with very few exceptions the predicted narrow therapeutic ratio and nature of the toxicities involved mean that the majority of potential anti-cancer drugs are not suitable for testing in perfectly fit people, but are first tested in patients who have cancer. That is easy – the difficult part is to explain the concept of risk with very little chance of benefit. I have sometimes been challenged by Ethics Committees as to whether there is *any* benefit for a patient who agrees to participate in a FIMS. Are we not merely exposing patients to potential toxicities at a most vulnerable time in the course of their disease if they have exhausted the known alternatives? The answer to this is a definite "no" – unquestionably there *are* benefits for patients taking part in these trials, but they are subtle.

When patients are told that they have run out of the known therapeutic options (or that there are none), the great majority are understandably saddened and depressed. Apart from the obvious anxiety that the next phase will be terminal illness, many are also concerned about being abandoned. They fear that you will no longer want to see them, that they will be told to go home and prepare for the inevitable – alone, or at least away from the specialist medical care to which they have grown accustomed. Whilst this anxiety may be completely misplaced, the opportunity to participate in a further trial – albeit where the medical profession is most likely to be the beneficiary – nevertheless offers a sense of purpose to their remaining life, and guarantees the continuing care and attention which can be so essential at this most vulnerable time in their whole illness. I have had many experiences where patients and relatives have genuinely expressed their gratitude for being able to be "useful", and to make a contribution to medical knowledge by taking part in a phase I/FIMS.

So when you have selected a patient for whom you think that participation in one of these trials is appropriate, you must explain the concept of very low doses, of exploration – indeed, the ultimate concept of the unfamiliar, or the unknown. At the same time you must emphasise that you will be taking every possible care to monitor organ function and every aspect of their health, in order to answer the scientific question without causing them any avoidable harm. However much you would wish a patient to participate, you must avoid any suggestion that the patient "ought" to participate, any suggestion that you will be disappointed if they decline, and above all any inappropriate promise of benefit – "miracles can happen", etc. Yet all of this must be explained within the concept of avoiding hopelessness – of letting the patient think that this is the last gasp. When inviting patients to consider a phase I/FIMS, I usually use the expression of "partnership": that if they wish to participate in this kind of trial, they will be joining us "as partners" in a clinical research study. I have found that this language can be received in a positive way – helping the patient to feel that indeed their lives are not yet over, that there are still elements of positivity that can ease the transition from the active and hopeful phases of treatment to the acceptance of terminal care, whilst avoiding or softening the feeling of hopelessness and abandonment once active treatment has finished.

Complementary and alternative medicine (CAM) is the term used to describe practices and products that are outside standard medical practice. The concept has been around for hundreds of years and of course far precedes modern cancer treatment, but the use of CAM has escalated dramatically in recent years and is now widely used – especially amongst cancer patients. The subject is controversial and, as well as being capable of unquestionable benefit for some patients, CAM can actually cause harm as well.

As an oncologist, it is not likely to be your primary responsibility to explain CAM, but you may be asked for your opinion about different aspects of this, and if your patient is using CAM there are significant advantages for them if they are made aware that you are comfortable to discuss this with them. As with so many aspects of communication referred to in the preceding sections of this book, the better you establish trust and communication with your patient, the better you are able to help them – with treatment choices, conventional or otherwise, and with coping with all the challenges that follow a diagnosis of cancer.

The term CAM includes a large number of different approaches that represent an alternative to conventional medicine. Various aspects of nutrition, diets and dietary supplements are widely promoted. Herbal medicines are amongst the oldest remedies that have been used, whilst physical therapies such as massage and yoga and psychological approaches such as relaxation techniques and hypnosis all have their supporters.

The concept of "integrative oncology" is an important development in recent years, where patients and practitioners are seeking to integrate CAM with conventional anti-cancer medicine. This is important, because it offers patients the opportunity to use CAM openly without fear of alienating their physician, it allows the latter to develop a more complete picture of their patient's health, cautioning where necessary about any negative effects of CAM, and above all it facilitates the possibility of conducting research, potentially to develop an evidence base for CAM – the lack of which creates the greatest difficulty for doctors.

It is not appropriate to discuss in detail the pros and cons of CAM in these pages, but it may be helpful to make a few general comments, particularly concerning benefit and risk.

When patients seek a discussion about CAM, they may be genuinely asking for your opinion about positives and potential negatives. They may on the other hand be testing you out, to see whether you approve or disapprove of unconventional practices. How you respond to such questions is entirely up to you and will depend on your own beliefs in the various strategies employed, but my advice is to try to avoid any sense of dismissing their interests and beliefs out of hand. Any suggestion by you that CAM is quirky, unscientific, unproven and therefore useless will only alienate your patient, and create an environment where your ability to help them with conventional therapy is diminished. This is not to say that you have to offer unreserved support – it is a question of balance. It is important to remember the reasons why people use CAM and to try to help them understand any potential harmful influences on their health which might arise from their use.

The two major reasons why patients seek the help of CAM are, firstly, their anxiety that conventional medicine cannot help them enough and, secondly, that they want to take some control of their lives at a time when they feel especially vulnerable and otherwise dependent.

We do not need to be shy about admitting the limitations of current anti-cancer treatments. As oncologists we are here to offer the best that there is and to explain the limits of benefit or otherwise in a coherent and honest fashion. Patients accept this, but if their particular prognosis is poor or they are greatly distressed by the uncertainties of their future, it is entirely understandable that they should seek any and all alternative approaches. If you engage your patients in frank conversation about this, you will enhance the trust they have in you, and you will be better informed about their attitude to conventional as well as CAM therapies. This is key, because there is no reason why CAM may not complement conventional medicine (with a few exceptions, see below), but as their oncologist you need a comprehensive picture of what your patient is experiencing and possibly experimenting with.

Regarding physical therapies – massage, relaxation, exercise – there are very few contraindications or concerns in terms of your management and advice. The only caveat to this is where occasionally patients may embark on extreme exercise regimes, which can exhaust them and cause actual harm – but this is rare.

Diets can be problematic. Many patients with cancer find nutrition a problem – weight loss resulting from cachexia can be confounded by alterations in taste, reduced levels of exercise, sleeplessness, constipation from analgesia, and a host of other factors all contributing to problems in maintaining a balanced and sufficiently nutritious diet. There are many specific diets advocated to help patients – some promoted to have actual anti-cancer benefits. These may involve focusing on specific additions to a normal diet (including vitamin supplements), or deleting foods, for example dairy produce or red meat. Notwithstanding the problem of creating sound, scientific evidence for or against these diets, it may be helpful for you to discuss the relative importance of such alterations in eating habits with your patients. Any encouragement that you can give to ensure a balanced diet can only be helpful, but – as with all discussions about CAM (remembering the reasons that patients embark on this) – it is more useful to be broadly supportive than critical. The only reason to counsel against this is if you suspect that the patient is actually harming their health in the case of diet, either by adopting some extreme diet that deprives them of basic nutrition or by causing them to obsess about their cancer in an unnatural way. I well remember the promotion of a particular antioxidant diet many years ago that required the patient to spend literally 4–5 hours a day preparing their special vegetable-based diet. This not only caused them to obsess about their cancer on a daily basis, but excluded many hours available for activity, especially involving their families, and was ultimately considered to definitely cause more harm than good.

Users of CAM often recount the benefit that they feel from "doing something for themselves" – from taking some control over their cancer. Such simple things as taking daily food supplements, enrolling in an exercise class, meditation or having regular massage can restore some sense that life is not out of control, and as doctors we should empathise with this.

So are there any downsides to CAM? Unfortunately, yes. Apart from dietary issues mentioned above, the biggest problem with CAM is the situation where patients are either so disillusioned with conventional medical approaches, or so seduced by the advertisements for CAM, that they abandon conventional medicine altogether. Given that modern oncology can help virtually everyone to some extent, this is obviously a sad situation. It is also potentially very difficult for a patient's family, who may then be torn between the wishes of their loved one but also, being more removed from the actual illness, wishing that routine approaches could be included as well. In this situation you may find yourself as a go-between and must try to steer both patient and family back from the extreme of rejecting conventional treatment to a compromise where both CAM and established medical approaches are used – indeed, this is the concept of "integrative oncology".

Apart from the situation of total rejection of conventional medicine and harm from extreme diets or exercise, there are some other proven negatives associated with CAM. Some substances taken as part of CAM may cause actual harm, either directly, by interfering with the immune system, or by specific drug interactions that can affect conventional medicines that you have prescribed.

One of the earliest examples of this is Laetrile, sometimes called vitamin B17, a substance chemically related to amygdalin, which occurs naturally in the stones of apricots. Amygdalin is digested to form hydrogen cyanide, explaining its toxicity! The history of this goes back over 100 years, but Laetrile received particular notoriety in the 1970s, leading to the National Cancer Institute (NCI) in the USA having to perform formal clinical trials. The latter not only reported no clinical benefit, but importantly reported significant cyanide-related toxicities.

Another compound that has attracted notoriety is St John's wort. St John's wort is a herbal medicine most often used as an antidepressant. It has been clearly shown that, through induction of cytochrome P450 enzymes, St John's wort reduces the plasma levels of a wide variety of conventional medicines including antibiotics, antidepressants, anticoagulants, digoxin, diuretics and various anti-cancer drugs. It is clearly important therefore that, if patients wish to avail themselves of St John's wort, their prescriber of conventional medicines is fully aware of this.

Your role as their medical oncologist is to counsel your patients about the holistic approach to cancer care. Your primary responsibility is their routine medical care and research, where appropriate, but in explaining the benefits and limitations of modern cancer medicine you will certainly on occasion be challenged to give your views on CAM. Whilst you may wish to be critical of the lack of scientific evidence for various CAM practices, I recommend that you avoid appearing critical of your patients' wish to seek all and every avenue that might help them.

Understanding their motivation may enable you to support the positive aspects of CAM whilst warning against extreme or bizarre practices, and especially proven negative or potentially harmful interactions.

The development of "integrative oncology" is, in my opinion, a positive step in trying to encourage the continuation of proven medical interventions with these alternative approaches. Attempts are being made to establish an evidence base, and major institutions such as the MD Anderson Cancer Center and the NCI in the USA are conducting clinical trials to address this. However, the greatest challenge is to design a trial that addresses only one aspect of CAM – either in comparison with conventional medicine or as an addition to this. Asking consenting patients to restrict themselves to only one specific aspect of CAM to the exclusion of all others is going to be difficult, to say the least. Nevertheless, as with so many aspects of modern cancer care referred to in these pages, open, honest and caring conversation is the key. If you can explain what modern medicine has to offer and listen to what your patient wants, hopes for, and is trying to accomplish, then you have done everything that is asked of you – and done it well.

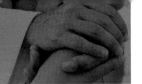

Epilogue

Looking after the doctor

The purpose of writing this book was to offer some advice about how to explain the complexities of cancer and its management to patients and their families. I have written it principally for young doctors embarking on a career in oncology, calling on my 40 years' experience in the field. I hope that some elements of this will help you to find your own way to conducting these delicate conversations, to offer intelligible explanations of multi-modal complex medicine to vulnerable anxious patients. Experience makes this easier – we all learn from our mistakes and hopefully build on the things that seem to work, but this is a very challenging practice within medicine. Within the total compass of medicine, oncology results remain poor, while the public and especially our patients' expectations remain high, and inevitably we have to deal with disappointment.

Oncology is challenging for everyone involved – especially you. Day after day you meet new patients, you have to try to explain their individual circumstances and options, and, as with every other aspect of professional life, there is repetition involved. All of us find it hard to offer the same level of compassion late on a Friday afternoon compared with first thing on a Monday morning! And so my final words of advice concern looking after yourself as the doctor. Giving out all the information referred to in these pages, inevitably involving yourself to some degree in your patient's distress, constantly being confronted with the disappointment of resistance, relapse, progressive disease, etc., takes its toll on the giver of the information, as well as the receiver.

There are many studies describing the concept of "burn-out" in oncologists, the time when the ability to keep giving of one's best is stretched to the limit and beyond. It is never too early in your career to be aware of the risk of "burn-out" and to devise strategies to avoid this. One relevant piece of advice is to share as much as possible with colleagues – your own peer group, your seniors and, in due course, those whom you train. Sharing your daily experience, your anxiety about a difficult decision, admitting to mistakes when a key conversation has gone wrong, sharing your sadness when a patient suffers a particularly unfair setback – these can free you from inappropriate self-criticism, and can truly "lighten your load". Always remember that by offering compassion, empathy and understanding, it is possible to help literally every patient who seeks your help – and it will be a very unusual day when you go home from the hospital, clinic or office not being able to reflect on genuinely having helped someone who was greatly distressed. Not all branches of medicine offer that.

Not long ago a medical student asked me how I dealt with "difficult" patients. I asked her what she meant by "difficult" and she replied, "Surely there must have been patients who you simply did not like". The answer was easy: it is not our role to categorise patients into those who we naturally like or dislike; we must offer the same empathy and concern to every patient who comes under our care. This does, however, remind me to offer a comment on patients with whom you identify in a very personal way – patients of your own age, patients who remind you of a parent or close relation, a fellow doctor or nurse. In looking after such patients, you need to take extra care with your own reactions, emotions and sympathies. Their disease, their suffering, is not your fault – and is only your responsibility in the strictest professional sense. Try to treat everyone in the same, constant way – but for this particular situation, anticipate that you may need extra support in order to maintain your own private equilibrium.

So my advice is to seek the company of your colleagues for professional support, and your friends and family for the essential recreation that, if you work at it, should allow you to switch off and recharge your personal batteries. Oncology is one of the hardest challenges within medicine, but it also brings great rewards – so pace yourself – and practice long enough to experience them!

Further Reading

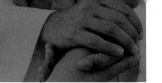

- *On Death and Dying.* E. Kübler-Ross.
  Toronto: Macmillan, 1969.

- *Difficult Conversations in Medicine.* E. Macdonald.
  Oxford: Oxford University Press, 2010.

- *When Cancer Crosses Disciplines.* M. Robotin, I. Olver and A. Girgis.
  London: Imperial College Press, 2010.

John Smyth is Emeritus Professor of Medical Oncology in the University of Edinburgh. He received his undergraduate training at Cambridge University and St Bartholomew's Hospital in London. He trained in Medical Oncology, initially under Professor Gordon Hamilton Fairley at St Bartholomew's and subsequently at the Royal Marsden and Institute of Cancer Research in London and at the National Cancer Institute (NIH), USA.

He was appointed to the Inaugural Chair of Medical Oncology in Edinburgh University in 1978, from which he retired in 2008. Over those 30 years he established Edinburgh as one of the major medical oncology centres in Europe, and locally created a comprehensive cancer centre including laboratory research with medical, radiation and surgical oncology together with palliative care, serving a population of 1.5 million people. He is a fellow of the Royal Colleges of Physicians of Edinburgh and London, a Fellow of the Royal College of Surgeons of Edinburgh, a Fellow of the Royal College of Radiology and a Fellow of the Royal Society of Edinburgh.

With a research focus on drug development, he has played a longstanding role with the European Organisation for Research and Treatment of Cancer (EORTC) as a Member of the Early Clinical Trials Group, the Founder Chairman of the Pharmacokinetics and Metabolism Group, and subsequently on their Board and Charitable Trust. He was President of ESMO from 1991–1993 and President of the Federation of European Cancer Societies from 2005–2007, which he transformed into the European CanCer Organisation (ECCO).

From 2000–2009 he was Editor in Chief of the *European Journal of Cancer*. He has to date published more than 320 papers and contributed to 46 books. He is married with two daughters, two step-daughters and four very energetic grandchildren!

Index